Dictionary of
medical equipment

Dictionary of
medical equipment

Malcolm Brown, BSc(Eng), PhD
Principal Physicist

Paul Hammond, BSc
Senior Physicist

Tony Johnson
Chief Technician

The Institute of Medical and Dental Bioengineering
Royal Liverpool Hospital
Liverpool
United Kingdom

LONDON

Chapman and Hall

First published in 1986 by
Chapman and Hall Ltd
11 New Fetter Lane, London EC4P 4EE

© 1986 M. Brown

Printed in Great Britain by
J.W. Arrowsmith Ltd, Bristol

ISBN 0 412 28290 9

British Library Cataloguing in Publication Data

Brown, Malcolm
    Dictionary of medical equipment.
    1. Medical instruments and apparatus ——
    Dictionaries
    I. Title II. Hammond, Paul III. Johnson,
    Anthony
    610'.28   R856.A3

    ISBN 0-412-28290-9

Preface

This dictionary was begun on the basis of the inventory of medical equipment maintained for Liverpool Health Authority, to provide a brief description of all the items in use. However, the list has been extended with the aid of the reference works listed at the the end of the book, and also as a result of comments received from readers of the draft text.

The object has been to provide rudimentary information about equipment which may be found in hospitals, and in medical research and teaching institutions. It is intended to be useful to all those concerned with the use, servicing, or purchasing of medical and scientific equipment.

There are many common terms and trade names which are used for medical equipment. These have only been included where we have found that the terms are frequently used, or, in the case of trade names, that the term is used to refer to a general type of equipment rather than just a single model. The descriptions of equipment are meant as a guide, and are not definitive specifications.

To assist the reader to make best use of the dictionary, Appendix 2 has been created to show entries listed according to subject. For instance, if an item found in a catalogue of medical equipment is not found in the dictionary, other relevant entries may be identified by examining the subject.

It is impossible to cover every item of equipment, and in any case, development, invention, and change in medical practice make it difficult to be truly up to date. However, we believe that all the commonly used items are covered, and that readers will find the information they require, in almost every case. Comments and suggestions, or information about difficulties in identifying equipment, will be gratefully received. The address to write to is The Institute of Medical and Dental Bioengineering, Royal Liverpool Hospital, Liverpool L7 8XP, in the United Kingdom.

Malcolm Brown

Acknowledgements

Special acknowledgement for assistance given during the writing of this dictionary must be given to the people listed below.

Dr Charles Chavasse of the Institute of Medical and Dental Bioengineering, University of Liverpool, for assistance with the text.

Dr Thien How, Lecturer in the Institute of Medical and Dental Bioengineering, University of Liverpool, for assistance with the ultrasound entries.

Mr Guy Lightfoot, Audiological Scientist at the Royal Liverpool Hospital, for assistance with the audiology entries.

Mrs Barbara Peattie, Senior Chief Physiological Measurement Technician, Cardio-respiratory Department, Royal Liverpool Hospital, for assistance with entries relating to cardiology.

Miss Gill Porter, District Speech Therapist, Liverpool Health Authority, for assistance with entries on speech therapy equipment.

Mr Douglas Redman, Senior Chief Technician in the Renal Dialysis Unit, Liverpool Health Authority, for assistance with entries relating to renal dialysis.

Mrs Vanessa Sluming of the School of Radiography, Liverpool, for assistance with entries relating to diagnostic X-ray equipment and ultrasound equipment.

Introduction

Supplementary information

Supplementary information is provided in coded form in the following way:

(e.g.) AUDIOMETER n=4 c=2,3,4 r=3

The coded information can be interpreted as follows:

n=4   A typical general hospital (with research and teaching functions) would have about four of these items.

c=2,3,4   These items are available in approximate price bands 2, 3 and 4.
          Price bands at date of writing given below are as follows
          1. 0   –   £100 ($150)
          2. £100   –   £500 ($750)
          3. £500   –   £1000 ($1500)
          4. £1000   –   £5000 ($7500)
          5. £5000   –   £10 000 ($15 000)
          6. £10 000   –   £50 000 ($75 000)
          7. £50 000   – £100 000 ($150 000)
          8. over £100 000 – (over ($150 000)

r=3   Extra information about this entry can be found in reference 3 at the end of the dictionary.

The following appendices are also included:

Appendix 1   List of abbreviations and acronyms

Appendix 2   List of entries by subject
               Anaesthesia
               Audiology and speech therapy
               Cardiology
               Dialysis
               Electrical, electronics and computing
               Lung function testing
               Ionizing radiation equipment
               Laboratory equipment
               Miscellaneous
               Physiotherapy
               Surgery
               Ultrasonics

Appendix 3   Useful literature

A-Scanner n=3 c=4 r=1

An ultrasonic scanning device employing ultrasonic pulses in the megahertz range is used to detect the depth of reflecting structures within the body. The distance into the body is displayed on the x-axis of a cathode ray tube (CRT) and the returning echoes are displayed as vertical movements (Y-axis), the echo amplitude being shown by the extent of the vertical movement. A-scanners were first used in the 1950s to detect the correct position of the 'midline echo' in the brain, which originates from the falx cerebri. Early A-scanners were converted industrial echo-sounders intended for detecting micro-cracks in metals.

Now, medical A-scanners exist which are intended purely for midline detection and incorporate 'swept gain' correction circuits to compensate for the attenuation of ultrasound which occurs in human tissue. These are used in the casualty or in the X-ray department as a cheap and non-invasive method of identifying the possible cause of concussion where this may be due to the existence of 'space occupying lesions' (tumours, haematomas, etc.) which may be displacing the midline from its normal position.

In addition many other ultrasonic scanners include an A-scan display to show that the 'swept gain' circuit is set correctly and to enable accurate distance measurements to be made between echoes. This measurement facility has proved particularly useful in the measurement of bi-parietal diameter (BPD) in the foetus to establish gestational age.

An A-scanner would normally consist of a single disc piezo electric damped transducer resonating at a chosen frequency between 2 and 15 MHz, a high voltage pulse generator to energize the transducer (at about 1 kHz), a tuned radio frequency amplifier, and the usual CRT drive circuitry. It is only really different from industrial versions by having a circuit to sweep the gain of the R.F. amplifier to compensate for absorption of the ultrasound in tissue.

Absorber n=20 c=2 r=2

Although this term could be applied to an acoustic or liquid absorber it is most commonly used to refer to a carbon dioxide absorber of the type used in rebreathing anaesthetic circuits. It consists of a container filled with

1

soda-lime through which the patient's expired gases are passed. It may take the form of a canister (e.g. Waters canister) mounted between the facepiece and breathing bag so that gas passes through in both directions, or it may be included in a circle closed circuit (see Circle absorber).

The soda-lime absorbs carbon dioxide from the expired gases so that the remainder can be fed back to the patient with a small supplement of fresh anaesthetic gases. This arrangement is economical with the gases used, reduces pollution of the room air, conserves heat and moisture, and does not normally require humidification. Disadvantages are that alkaline dust may pass to the patient, and the canister holding the granules may be a cause of leaks.

The soda-lime usually consists of a mixture of 90% calcium hydroxide, 5% sodium hydroxide, and 1% potassium hydroxide, with silicates to prevent powdering. It is essential for effective operation that moisture (14–19%) be incorporated within the granules. Durasorb is an improved soda-lime which is pink in colour which turns to white when it becomes inactive.

Absorption spectrometer n=1 c=4 r=9

Various chemicals whether in the gas or liquid phase absorb energy from specific regions of the electromagnetic radiation spectrum. Thus infrared radiation passed through two parallel chambers to a detection device may be used to record the difference in infrared absorption. The difference is sometimes detected in a Golay cell which consists of two infrared absorption chambers separated by a diaphragm whose movement is detected by a capacitance change with respect to an adjacent electrode. The infrared radiation is passed through a chopping disc so that each cell in turn receives the radiation causing alternating displacement of the diaphragm in the Golay cell. The diaphragm will be displaced to one side or other depending on the relative quantities of infrared light reaching the absorption chambers. An electronic circuit to amplify, demodulate and linearize the output is connected to the capacitance transducer.

One of the cells is filled with a reference gas while the other is filled with a background gas plus a small flow-through of the gas being sampled. The modification in absorption is used to detect the molar fraction of the sample gases. Problems arise where the absorption spectra of the gases being tested overlap (e.g. nitrous oxide and halothane, carbon dioxide and carbon monoxide). The device requires a long stabilization period and the results will be affected by changes in atmospheric pressure.

Such instruments can be used for the analysis of gases in the lung function laboratory. They may also be called gas chromatographs.

Acoustic booth n=2 c=5 r=8

In hospitals this normally takes the form of a small room or chamber in which audiometric tests are performed. The DHSS (UK) recommendations for the design of ENT departments states that for such tests the maximum ambient noise is 30 dBA and the maximum reverberation time is 250 ms. This can be achieved by suitable construction and treatment of a room or preferably by the installation of an acoustically isolated inner chamber. Acoustic booths found in many hospitals do not meet these standards, and other requirements such as wheelchair access and silent ventilation have often been neglected.

Other names for an acoustic booth may include sound-proof room, audiometric room and anechoic chamber (although this term normally applies to a research installation with more stringent specifications).

Acoustic impedance meter/bridge n=2 c=4 r=3

A device for measuring the integrity of the sound conduction mechanism between the ear drum and the oval window to the inner ear by measuring the acoustic impedance of the ear drum. In the normal ear, sound applied to the ear drum will readily pass through,and a low acoustic impedance is measured. If sound will not pass through easily (due to a defect in the middle ear) then a high acoustic impedance may be recorded. The acoustic impedance is recorded while varying the pressure in the outer ear (typically from +2 kPa to −6 kPa). A minimum impedance is recorded when the pressure in the outer ear is the same as that in the middle ear (i.e. where there is no pressure differential across the ear drum causing it to stiffen), thus allowing the middle ear air pressure to be measured indirectly. In the normal case the middle ear pressure is close to atmospheric whereas in many pathological conditions it is lower.

For clinical use in the ENT or audiology department, the measurements are recorded on an X–Y plotter (which may be part of the acoustic impedance meter) on which the Y-axis shows compliance (the inverse of impedance) expressed in equivalent air volume (e.g. 0–4 ml), and the X-axis shows air pressure applied to the outer ear.

The apparatus normally consists of a low-pressure air pump and the necessary controls, a sound source and ear piece, an oscillator (usually about 220 Hz), and an amplifier and metering circuit. The unit may contain or be connected to an X–Y plotter.

Actinotherapy apparatus r=10

This term is synonymous with radiotherapy apparatus but its use in medical work is normally limited to equipment delivering electromagnetic radiations up to the ultraviolet range, and is most commonly applied to phototherapy. In some definitions actinotherapy relates to chemical changes brought about by radiation therapy but in physiotherapy this aspect is not usually stressed since the therapy is mainly intended to impart heat to the tissues. See also Short-wave diathermy, Phototherapy, Infrared lamp, and Ultraviolet treatment unit.

Active electrode r=4 c=1 r=4

This is an electrosurgery electrode used for cutting or coagulation of tissue. It may be in the shape of a knife, needle, ball or loop. The electrodes with a small contact area with the tissue are used for cutting and excising sections of tissue, employing the cutting action of high-frequency (0.5-4 MHz) continuous wave currents. Electrodes with large surface areas are used for coagulation, drawing sparks from high-voltage pulses on to the tissue to arrest bleeding.

Acupuncture apparatus n=1 c=3,4

Various items of equipment exist for the acupuncturist. These include electrical stimulators, electrical impedance meters, and low-power infrared lasers. The electrical impedance meter is used to locate low impedance points on the skin, which are thought to correspond to acupuncture points. The electrical stimulators are similar to other low-power types used for pain relief and may be used to apply electrical stimulation to the acupuncture points via needles, or via point or plate electrodes. Low-power lasers are used to stimulate the acupuncture points and are claimed to have similar therapeutic effects.

Such devices might be found in the physiotherapy department or in an acupuncture or pain relief clinic.

ADC/DAC interface

Electrical signals from a piece of medical laboratory equipment or clinical equipment may be processed by a digital computer and returned to an analogue output device (e.g. pen recorder) using an ADC/DAC. The ADC (analogue to digital converter) examines incoming voltage at regular intervals (e.g. every microsecond up to every second) and converts the voltage to a binary number. The computer can then use this binary number or a series of them to make calculations and to identify trends. The results of the calculations can be returned to the output device through a digital to analogue converter (DAC) which produces a voltage representing the binary number given by the computer.

Many medical instruments incorporate ADCs and DACs without any external presentation of the digital form in which the calculations are performed. If a commercial computer or microcomputer is used then an external device may be required to perform these functions. In this case the computer controls the sampling rate and timing of the calls for the input of information and meets the requirement for timing and scaling of the output information.

Air bed n=5 c=3,4

Patients who are immobile for long periods may develop pressure sores. These can be avoided by repeatedly moving the patient so that different parts of the skin are supporting the body weight. An alternative method is to use a ripple bed/mattress which can be water or air filled. The air-filled types have an air pump which alternately inflates and deflates cells in the mattress over a period of a few minutes (e.g. 10 minutes).

Air embolus detector r=9

Whenever fluids are infused into the blood stream it is important to prevent the passage of air into the body. Air bubbles are undesirable and a large quantity of air reaching the heart can interfere with its pumping action.

All devices which could cause air to pass into the body should employ warning and fail-safe circuits to prevent this happening. The problem is most important in the use of infusion pumps where a disconnection or exhaustion of the fluid reservoir could lead to the pumping of air. Also when blood is removed from the body for oxygenation or dialysis it is essential that blood is returned to the body free from air bubbles.

There are two main types of air embolus detector which may be separate devices or incorporated into the parent instrument. These employ optical transmission, providing a warning when there is a sudden change in transmission. Alternatively, an ultrasonic device may be employed and this may also be monitoring the flow velocity within the tube if it is carrying blood. Doppler ultrasonic flow-meters calculate the blood velocity from the back-scattered ultrasound from the blood corpuscles. Air bubbles produce echoes which are several orders of magnitude greater in intensity than is received from the blood. The appearance of these very large echoes is used to identify the presence of air in the tube. Very small bubbles can be detected by this method.

Air entrainment valve

Also called an air inspiratory valve, this comprises a knife-edge seat, a disc and spring, and operates in an anaesthetic breathing circuit in the opposite way to a pressure relief valve, i.e. for the valve to open it requires a very small negative pressure to be exerted which causes the disc to lift allowing air to be entrained. The entrainment valve would operate if the patient was in spontaneous respiration and there was an obstruction in the fresh gas to the patient (e.g. a kink in the gas feed tube), or after the operation of an oxygen failure warning device which cuts off the the gases. Entrainment valves are incorporated in some anaesthetic machines, ventilators, and oxygen failure devices.

Air Viva respirator/resuscitator c=1 r=2

This is a bag, expiratory valve and facepiece for emergency resuscitation. The bag is inflated in its resting state so that after squeezing to inflate the lungs it automatically re-inflates with fresh air. Oxygen may be fed in via a narrow tube and a small valve. It is generally similar to the Ambu resuscitator.

Airway r=4

This normally refers to a device (tube) to keep the tongue from blocking airflow to the lungs during resuscitation, anaesthesia, or positive pressure ventilation. It may be passed through the nose (nasopharyngeal airway), the mouth (oropharyngeal airway) or through a tracheostomy.

AIUM test object n=1 c=2 r=1

This is a device for testing the performance of ultrasonic scanners and consists of two parallel plates of Perspex between which there are a number of steel or nylon threads. It may be a closed system containing a fluid with a velocity of sound transmission equal to that of tissue (usually 1540 m/s) or it may be an open frame intended to be immersed in a bath of suitable fluid. This fluid can be a special mixture of ethyl alcohol in water at room temperature or water may be warmed to 47°C at which the transmission velocity is correct.

There are four rows of wires in the frame as follows:

1. A row of equally spaced wires down the frame to give an indication of variation of the ultrasonic beam width with depth, and also of sensitivity with depth.
2. A row of wires across the frame at the bottom.
3. A row of wires across the frame close to the transducer which are spaced equally but each successive wire is slightly further away from the transducer. These indicate the depth of the transmit artefact or deadzone

due to the ringing of the transducer after the transmit pulse has been sent.
4. A row of wires moving progressively away from the transducer position which have progressively smaller spaces between them to demonstrate axial resolution.

The AIUM is the American Institute for Ultrasound in Medicine.

Aldasorber n=40 c=1

Anaesthetic gases and vapours released into the atmosphere in operating departments are thought to be harmful to the health or performance of those who work there. Measures to reduce air pollution are being implemented including better air conditioning, scavenging of the exhaled gases during anaesthesia and ducting these away, more frequent use of closed anaesthetic circuits, and the use of absorbers and adsorbers for anaesthetic vapours.

The Aldasorber is one type of these which adsorbs halothane and other vapours. It is disposable, and is changed when the weight has increased by a specified amount.

Ambu 'E' valve c=1 r=2

This is an expiratory valve for use in an anaesthetic breathing circuit which has been designed to prevent the passage of expired gases back into the breathing circuit and reservoir bag. Unintentional rebreathing of expired gases is a problem when using the conventional Magill circuit for controlled or assisted ventilation. The reservoir bag, being empty at the end of inspiration, tends to fill partially with expired gas during the expiratory phase. The Ambu 'E' valve is a two-stage valve fitted in place of the usual expiratory valve which makes sure that expired gases are directed out of the breathing circuit altogether. The Ruben's valve is intended to achieve the same result but with slightly different construction.

Ambu facepiece c=1 r=2

A type of facemask for anaesthesia which has a transparent body allowing early detection of vomit, which is particularly useful during resuscitation. This type also has an inflatable sealing cuff to improve the fit on to the face.

Ambu respirator/resuscitator c=1 r=2

For providing emergency artificial respiration for resuscitation this consists of a bag, valve and facepiece. The bag remains inflated in its resting state and when squeezed closes the expiratory port and inflates the patient's lungs. When the bag is released it automatically re-inflates with fresh air and the patient's expired air passes out to atmosphere via the expiratory valve. Oxygen may be supplied to the bag via a small tube and valve at one end of the bag. The facepiece is usually transparent so that vomit can be seen. A similar type of respirator is the Air Viva.

Ambulatory ECG monitor n=2 c=5 r=3

Abnormalities of the ECG and heart rate may not show when the patient is being monitored in the clinic. At one time it was common to confine the patient to bed and watch the ECG tracing for a few days. Automatic monitors are now available which will recognize abnormalities in the cardiac rhythm.

A special type of automatic arrhythmia detector monitors the patient during his normal working day by means of a special cassette tape recorder which is carried by the patient under investigation. By suitable data compression mechanisms the whole 24 hours (approximately 100 000 heart beats) can be compressed on to one cassette and this is read through on the following day at high speed to identify the frequency and significance of fluctuations in the heart rhythm.

The whole apparatus consists of a number of special portable tape recorders complete with ECG leads and electrodes, and the arrhythmia analyser which is kept at the hospital. The analyser consists of a cassette playback mechanism and a small computer programmed to recognize variations in the heart rate, and possibly abnormalities of the ECG itself. Typically, the output would be a histogram of the heart rate over the 24 hours and the ability to reproduce small sections of the ECG waveform relating to unusual events.

The use of such apparatus is much more cost efficient than long-term monitoring in the coronary intensive care unit, and is also more likely to detect transitory problems because the patient is performing normal tasks.

Anaesthetic Circuit r=2

The part of an anaesthetic machine which contains gases at low (near atmospheric) pressure. This includes all components on the back bar, and the breathing circuit. It does not include the cylinders, pipelines and the various high-pressure control components.

Anaesthetic machine n=40 c=4 r=2

Sometimes referred to as the anaesthetic trolley, this normally refers to a trolley on which are mounted gas cylinders and/or pipelines for various gases used in anaesthesia, together with the various valves, controls and ancillary equipment used by the anaesthetist.

8

These are found in all operating theatres and also in special procedure rooms in the X-ray department, accident and emergency unit, dental clinics and some community clinics. On the trolleys, the gases can be dispensed and mixed. These usually include oxygen, nitrous oxide and carbon dioxide, and sometimes medical air, cyclopropane and anaesthetic vapours such as halothane, ether, etc. The vapours are usually provided in special vaporizers which may be interchangeable according to the particular anaesthetic procedure required.

Simpler machines may also be referred to as anaesthetic machines which only dispense a mixture of nitrous oxide and oxygen. These may be controllable devices such as the Walton 5 or operate from premixed bottled gases (Entonox unit). These latter may be used either on the ward or as a portable unit in ambulances or by district midwives. An anaesthetic machine may also be used in conjunction with, or be incorporated into, a ventilator.

The maintenance of such equipment requires especially formal arrangements and quality control measures, since incorrect operation may cause permanent injury to the patient.

The main components of an anaesthetic machine are high-pressure gas reservoirs and/or pipelines, pressure reducing valves, flowmeters (usually of the rotameter type), pressure gauges, carbon dioxide absorbers, a fresh gas outlet, oxygen flush assembly, and vaporizers. The trolley may also carry monitoring equipment such as ECG and pressure monitors, oxygen meters, oscillotonometer, temperature gauges and pulse monitors, and a Wright's respirometer. Some modern ventilators are also carried on the trolley and become an integral part of the anaesthetic circuit when in use. Other important parts of the system are the suction apparatus and gas scavenging devices.

Analgesia apparatus n=10 c=3 r=2

This is usually an intermittent demand flow machine for delivering a mixture of nitrous oxide and oxygen, possibly with an analgesic vapour during labour, emergency surgery or dentistry. Examples are the Entonox apparatus, Minnitt's apparatus (obsolete), McKesson, Lucy Baldwyn, Walton 5, AE, and Quantiflex RA.

Anechoic chamber n=0 c=6 r=8

This is a special room or chamber with very low ambient noise and reverberation characteristics used for acoustical or audiological testing in research establishments. The term is sometimes wrongly applied to audiometry rooms or acoustic booths used in hospitals. Acoustic booths have less stringent specifications for an installation of the same size.

Anemometer r=2

A device for measuring the velocity of a gas or liquid. The three common types are those which monitor the difference in pressure between two points in a duct (Venturi or Fleisch tube), those which detect the cooling effect of the flow past a heated body (hot wire anemometer), and those in which the flow drives a small windmill. An example of the latter type is the Wright's respirometer.

Aneroid pressure gauges n=50 c=1 r=2

An aneroid pressure gauge or manometer is used to measure relatively low pressure differences from atmospheric pressure. It consists of a metal (usually copper) cylinder with thin corrugated sides often seen in barometers. The cylinder contains air and is completely sealed so that changes in the external pressure cause it to become longer or shorter. One end of the cylinder is fixed, while the other connects to a rack and pinion, with a pointer attached to the pinion. The pointer thus moves over a scale indicating pressure. The system can also be used in reverse so that the pressure to be measured is fed to the inside of the cylinder. There will however be a small error due to changes in atmospheric pressure.

Antistatic chain r=2

Trolleys used in conjunction with anaesthetic apparatus are often seen to have a small metal chain hanging down and dragging on the floor. The object of this is to prevent the build-up of static electricity on the trolley which might otherwise cause sparking when connection is made between the equipment on the trolley and other metalwork. The sparks may in turn ignite anaesthetic gases or vapours.

The chain is not normally necessary because trolley wheels on anaesthetic equipment are usually made of antistatic (conductive) rubber which performs the same function.

Antistatic floor n=15 c=4 r=2

Sparks due to static electricity in operating theatres may cause ignition of spirits, or explosion. Also the small electric shocks received from these sparks may cause minor mishaps. To prevent the build-up of static electricity, the whole operating area is maintained at earth potential by the use of flooring materials which provide a limited leakage path for electricity. Sometimes the whole floor is covered with an antistatic rubber or plastic but satisfactory results can be obtained with tile floors (e.g. quarry, terrazzo) though these may depend on a high relative humidity in the room. Since operating theatres are normally maintained at a relative humidity of 50-65%, this condition is normally met.

Test criteria exist in some countries such as the requirement that the resistance between two electrodes 60 cm apart on the floor should be between 20 kΩ and 5 MΩ. The reason for the lower limit is that a very low resistance floor would present an enhanced risk of electrocution from faulty equipment or wiring by improving the potential current route to earth.

Antistatic rubber r=2

Rubber or Neoprene can be made into rather poor conductors of electricity by the addition of carbon. The poor conductivity achieved is ideal for use in the operating theatre for the construction of anaesthetic equipment tubing, operating table mats, floors and trolley wheels. Static electricity induced on to the surface of these items will leak away safely, thus reducing the risk of electrical sparks which may cause ignition of volatile anaesthetic agents. Items made of antistatic rubber are normally identified by a yellow flash or label.

Apnoea alarm/monitor n=20 c=2 r=2,3

This device monitors breathing and sounds an alarm if no breathing is detected for more than a preset time limit (e.g. 15-30 s). The two main applications for such devices are monitoring the breathing of premature babies and monitoring the correct action of ventilators in the operating theatre and intensive care unit.

An apnoea alarm for use on babies may operate in one of several ways:

1. Impedance plethysmography in which the electrical impedance of the chest is measured via skin electrodes. The impedance falls as the chest expands and so a signal roughly corresponding to the breathing pattern is obtained. This signal is applied to a circuit to identify when chest movement is insufficient to indicate breathing. In its simplest form this might be a rectifier, integrator and level detector which alarms if the voltage falls below a preset level. The whole device may be incorporated into an ECG monitor using the same electrodes.
2. Chest wall movement detectors may be used which detect the expansion in the chest circumference during breathing. These may be simple strain gauges included in a thread or tape around the chest, or mercury in elastic tubes which varies in electrical resistance as the tube is stretched. The term 'pneumograph' is often used to describe a wider bore air-filled tube

11

around the chest in which the pressure will vary with the breathing movement.

3. General movement of the infant may be a suitable substitute for actual chest wall movement since the apnoeic episodes experienced by young babies are normally associated with cessation of all movement. This may be detected with a crude form of radar device which directs a 10 GHz electromagnetic wave at the baby and detects changes in the phase of the returning echo and converts this into an activity signal to trigger the apnoea detecting circuit.

4. Movement may also be detected by a variety of sensing systems such as a pressure mattress using thermocouples to detect the flow of air which occurs between segments of an air mattress during movement, or a small air-filled bulb may be taped to the abdomen of the baby and the variations of pressure in the bulb be detected.

Ventilator alarms may monitor the source of power (gas or electricity) to the ventilator and will monitor pressure or flow in the breathing circuit. Typically they are set to alarm if the pressure exceeds a given value and if the cycling of pressure ceases for more than a preset interval. This type, which works in the breathing circuit, is preferable since it will also alarm if there is a disconnection. Examples of ventilator alarms are the Blease, and the East Ventilarm.

Applanation tonometer n=1 c=1,5 r=6,9

The pressure within an elastic-walled sphere or cylinder such as the eye, an artery, or the pregnant uterus can be measured from outside the walls by the use of an applanation tonometer. This may be a mechanical device consisting of a flat ring in which there is a concentric disc maintained flush with the surface of the outer ring but connected to a force transducer. When a section of the wall is flattened by the device the pressure required on the central disc to keep the wall flat is equal to the pressure within the sphere or cylinder. The pressure is calculated as the force applied divided by the area of the inner disc. Large devices of this type are commonly used to measure the intra-uterine pressure during labour. This device is sometimes called a tocodynamometer or guard ring tocograph, and the measuring instrument called a cardiotocograph, which also records heart rate. Smaller devices have been used for measuring pressures within arteries and also within the eye by direct application to the cornea.

A non-contact applanation tonometer exists for measuring intra-ocular pressures. Flattening of a small section of the cornea is achieved by a blast of air with force increasing linearly with time. Applanation is detected optically by shining a collimated light beam on to the test section on the cornea and detecting the reflection. As the cornea becomes flattened the light intensity received reaches a maximum as the cornea becomes a plane mirror. The whole operation takes a few milliseconds which avoids the need for medication or any effects from blink responses. A computer is normally used to control the air blast and to identify the timing of the peak light intensity. Such devices are used in the ophthalmology department.

A carotid pulse transducer used in timing of the left ventricular ejection time may also be a small applanation tonometer.

Applicator r=3

Apart from the obvious meaning of this word it is used for a device fitted to teletherapy apparatus in the radiotherapy department which fixes the spacing between the X-ray source and the patient. It mounts on to the X-ray or gamma head and may have parallel steel walls, or conical lead-lined walls, with or without a Perspex end-piece. The device will also define the width of the treatment beam.

Such devices are found in radiotherapy departments.

Ardran-Crooks cassette n=1 c=3,4 r=7

This is a special X-ray film cassette which produces a pattern on the X-ray film caused by the differing attenuations through various thicknesses of copper in the cassette. The pattern produced allows calculation of the kilovoltage of the X-ray set.

A general term for this device is a penetrameter, and more details are given under that heading.

Arrhythmia detector n=2 c=4 r=3

Some forms of heart disease are characterized by variations in the time between successive heart beats. In extreme cases this can mean completely missed beats, or extra (ectopic) beats occurring between two otherwise normal beats.

Identifying these abnormalities used to be performed by inviting the patient to come into the coronary intensive care unit and have a skilled nurse watch a cardioscope display of the ECG for several days.

This is a task ideally suited to computer pattern recognition programs and such devices are now available which detect these abnormalities and store the key elements of the information (e.g. reproducing a short strip of the ECG record relating to each abnormal event).

There have been various generations of machines to detect arrhythmias ranging from tape loops or multi-head tape recorders which compared the timing between the incoming beats with those of a few seconds before, to full pattern recognition systems which identify ectopic beats not only from their abnormal time relationship to the main beats but also because the shape of the ECG is different.

A new and most important variant on arrhythmia detectors is the ambulatory monitoring schemes utilizing small tape recorders which collect 24 hours of the patient's ECG during normal daily tasks. The cassette tape record of each day's activity is read through a computer-type analyser at high speed the following day. Various derived indices of the behaviour of the heart rate can be produced and in some cases abnormalities of the ECG itself can be identified.

Arrhythmia detectors and monitors will be found in the coronary intensive care unit, possibly in the intensive therapy unit and in one or two high dependency units in the medical wards.

Arterio-angiography apparatus $n=1$ $c=7,8$ $r=4$

For X-ray visualization of the larger arteries (e.g. coronary, cerebral, renal, femoral, aorta, etc.) it is usual to inject a bolus of contrast medium from a high-pressure syringe, into the artery itself. The progress of the contrast medium through the arterial system is then observed by fluoroscopy, usually backed-up by X-ray films produced by cine, or in a rapid film changer. The X-ray set may be a general set plus accessories, or may be dedicated equipment (single and bi-plane).

The apparatus used for this is an X-ray set with a fluoroscopic screen coupled to a video imaging system. A special high-pressure pump is also required to inject the dye in a short time to provide an identifiable bolus which will pass through the vessels.

Arteriosonde $n=3$ $c=4$

This is in fact a trade name for a version of an ultrasonic blood pressure meter or monitor. It is claimed to produce a measure of the systolic and diastolic blood pressure using a cuff on the arm which is more reliable and less subject to movement artefact than is achieved using acoustic or pulse monitoring techniques. It may be found anywhere in the hospital where blood pressures are taken and may include its own pen recorders to display the trend of pressure.

The mode of operation is to detect the movement of the arterial wall under the cuff on the arm by an ultrasonic doppler technique. The movements so detected are interpreted to display the required pressures. Before use, an ultrasonic coupling gel must be applied to the transducer elements to ensure adequate transmission of the ultrasound.

The main components of the machine are a pressure cuff for the arm, an inflation and control mechanism (the inflation and deflation are usually automatic), a continuous wave ultrasonic transmitter, transducer (separate elements for transmit and receive), ultrasonic receiver amplifier and doppler detector, discriminator and display and/or recording device. The recording device can also be programmed to operate at set intervals.

Arteriovenous shunt r=3,4

For haemodialysis blood must be removed from the body, passed through a dialyser and returned. Since it may be necessary to make and break these connections several times a week various methods have been developed for inserting tubes into blood vessels. The arteriovenous shunt consists of two PTFE (Teflon) and silicon rubber tube sets, one of which is connected into a tied-off artery and the other into a tied-off vein, usually at the wrist or lower leg. The silicon rubber tubes are brought out through the skin and are normally connected together, thereby forming a shunt between the artery and the vein. When haemodialysis is performed the connection is undone and blood from the artery will pass through the dialyser and back to the vein. These shunts are convenient to use but have proved relatively troublesome in terms of clotting, and infection at the site of passage through the skin.

Arteriovenous shunts have been largely supplanted by arteriovenous fistulae. In these cases an artery and a vein are tied off, each is slit for a few centimetres along each side and the two holes so created are sewn together, forming an internal shunt for the blood. The venous section bulges under the enlarged pressure providing a bulb of blood which is flowing rapidly, and can be easily penetrated by a wide bore needle or needles for haemodialysis. These fistulae have proved less troublesome than shunts.

Arthroscope n=1 c=3,4

This is a special endoscope for direct wide-angle viewing in bone joints.

Artificial artery r=4

The growing incidence of arterial disease, and improvements in diagnostic and treatment techniques have increased the demand for prosthetic vascular grafts, although the use of natural grafts (usually veins) is preferred where possible.

Prosthetic grafts should be seamless, have low porosity to blood, permit suturing, and be flexible but not kink.

Most existing arterial prostheses are woven or knitted and are corrugated to control kinking. However, these features disturb blood flow patterns which may cause blood clotting and deposition of other materials leading to the obstruction of the lumen.

Newer designs attempt to solve some of the these problems by the use of smooth tubing of biocompatible materials which may permit the growth of a more natural lining of the tube with consequent improvement in their long-term performance.

Artificial Ear n=1 c=2 r=8

When testing the sound pressure level generated by an earphone a coupling device is required between the earphone and the microphone of the sound pressure level meter which will simulate the acoustic impedance (effective compliance) of the natural ear. This normally takes the form of a cavity with correct fittings at each end for the earphone and the microphone and has a volume roughly equivalent to the ear/earphone system. For a normal earphone this volume us usually 6 ml and a simple device (called a 6 cc coupler) may be used, and for an ear plug or ear mould 2 ml is required (2 cc coupler). Simple couplers do not accurately simulate the impedance of a real ear and a true artificial ear has additional cavities in order to create the more complex impedance characteristics of a real ear.

Artificial ears are used in the calibration of hearing aids or headphones on their own or as part of an audiometer.

Artificial heart r=4

Although animal experiments involving total replacement of heart function have been conducted over several years, human experiments are relatively rare. The usual mechanism is to have a flexible diaphragm driven by a pneumatic control system.

Artificial heart valve r=4

All four valves in the heart can become diseased either restricting the flow (stenosis) or leaking backwards (insufficiency or regurgitation).

Over 200000 mechanical and tissue valves have been implanted in humans and there are three main types. These are:

1. Ball and cage valves such as the Smeloff.
2. Hingeless tilting disc valves such as the Bjork-Shiley.
3. Tissue valves employing animal tissue such as the valve taken from a specially bred pig.

In each case the valve is mounted on a sewing ring made of metal or plastic sheathed in woven fabric (usually Dacron) which is sewn into the orifice created by excising the natural valve. No artificial valve is a perfect substitute for the natural valve and the design requires a trade off of various factors to achieve the optimum solution.

The valve may restrict the flow to some extent, and allow more regurgitation than is desirable, and so the largest possible valve is used in the space available. The use of synthetic materials causes damage to the blood and long-term anticoagulant therapy is always necessary. The life of the valve is limited by fatigue and corrosion and this may be exacerbated by poor materials and poor design leading to excessive stresses in the structure or turbulence in the blood.

Considerable effort has been expended in the testing of artificial valves to optimize these factors. They are usually tested in heart simulators, sometimes called pulse duplicators, which employ a Perspex model of the heart with the valves mounted in it and a pump which generates a pulsatile flow driving a viscous liquid with similar mechanical properties to real blood.

Tissue valves require special treatment to ensure sterility and minimal antigenic reaction from the body.

Artificial kidney n=10 c=1,4 r=3,4

This is the dialyser as used in haemodialysis. It basically consists of a semipermeable membrane having pores about 500 nm in diameter. Molecules with molecular weight of less than 5000 can diffuse fairly easily through these pores; molecules of 500 to 40 000 molecular weight will pass more slowly, whereas larger molecules are restrained. Blood is passed along one side of the membrane while a special dialysate solution is passed along the other. The dialysate solution contains molecules which are not required to be withdrawn from the blood so that only unwanted molecules will diffuse from the blood into the dialysate. Also the dialysate may contain molecules to be passed to the blood and the concentration or pressure may be such as to withdraw water from the body.

There are three main types of artificial kidney: the coil dialyser in which the membranes are wound round in a spiral (this type is no longer used), the plate or parallel flow dialyser in which the blood and the dialysate flow on either side of large flat membranes (e.g. the Kiil dialyser), or there may be several parallel plates, and the hollow fibre dialyser, in which the membrane is made as many parallel small tubes. The Kiil dialyser is reusable except for the membranes and must be assembled and sterilized before each use. Other types are normally disposable or may be reused a few times following a regeneration and sterilization programme.

The term 'artificial kidney' is often applied to the whole system including the pumps and control circuitry for the dialysate mixing and delivery, and for the blood preparation and monitoring, pumping, de-aerating and return to the body.

Artificial larynx n=10 c=1,2 r=4

Where the larynx has been surgically removed, typically due to cancer, it is impossible to produce the vibrating sound necessary for speech. An artificial larynx is a vibrating source to provide air vibrations similar to the normal larynx. By the normal use of the mouth and tongue intelligible speech can be produced.

There are three main types of this device:

1. After tracheostomy air may be forced through a special device to create vibrations similar to those made by the normal larynx, and this air may be piped to the artificial opening in the neck to allow articulation in the mouth.
2. An electronic generator operating through a tube placed into the mouth can produce a similar effect.
3. The most common type in use at present is a small hand-held vibrator which is pressed against the neck or face so that vibrations are transmitted into the airway. This is rather like using an electric shaver pressed against the neck, and allows the user to carry on conversations or speak over the telephone. The speech is understandable but sounds artificial.

Artificial lung n=0 c=4 r=2

One would expect this term to be applied to devices for oxygenating the blood as used during cardiac bypass operations. However, the term has been coined to apply to forced ventilation of the lungs and in particular those machines which act by applying pressure to the chest externally such as the cabinet-type ventilator ('iron lung'), the cuirass or the Pinkerton cuirass ventilators. Such machines are no longer commonly found in acute hospitals.

Artificial mastoid n=1 c=3 r=8

An artificial mastoid is a device used to test the performance and calibration of the bone conduction transducer (vibrator) found on some hearing aids and most audiometers. The device itself consists of an accelerometer embedded in a mass approximating to that of the human skull, and is connected to a sound level meter or similar equipment used for the calibration of audiometers.

The transducer is held in contact with the accelerometer by a force of typically 540 grams and the face of the accelerometer has layers of rubber to simulate the compliance of the skin-covered mastoid bone (behind the ear) on which most bone conduction transducers are placed.

18

Artificial nose n=10 c=1 r=2

An ingenious condenser-humidifier is sometimes used during anaesthesia or artificial ventilation, which consists of a series of wire meshes in a metal housing. As the patient exhales, water vapour is condensed on the relatively cool wire mesh. During subsequent inhalation the vapour is re-evaporated and delivered to the lungs. They do not work very well and increase the dead space of the breathing circuit.

Artificial thumb

In paediatric anaesthesia it is common to use a breathing circuit of the Jackson-Rees T-piece configuration in which a small breathing bag is squeezed by the hand while occluding the open end between the finger and thumb. This provides a partial rebreathing of the gases contained in the connecting tubing. Electromechanical devices exist to provide the occlusion automatically and these are sometimes called artificial thumbs.

Aspirator r=2

This is a general term for a suction apparatus intended for drawing off mucus, saliva, blood, vomit, etc. into a reservoir. Various types of aspirator may be found listed under suction machine, suction unit, piped vacuum service, etc. They are used extensively in operating theatres and wards to drain operation sites and to clear the airways to prevent choking.

Atomic absorption spectrometer n=1 c=4 r=5,9

This is a form of flame photometer which measures the absorption of particular wavelengths of light when passing through a flame in which atoms from metal salts (e.g. sodium and potassium) are being ionized. Small samples of body fluids are aspirated into a nebulizer and injected into a flame of propane or natural gas, or into a flameless electrothermal arc (e.g. carbon rod furnaces). Light is passed through the flame generated by a hollow cathode lamp lined with a coating of the metal to be analysed. The characteristic spectral lines of the metal in question are radiated from the lamp and partially absorbed in the flame. A photometer detecting the radiation passing out of the flame can measure the quantity absorbed. Light emitted in the flame is separated from that absorbed, by pulsing the light source.

Although many metals may be determined in this way, calcium, magnesium, and lead, are the most common in the clinical chemistry department.

Atomizer r=2

A liquid may be broken up into small particles in a gas (an aerosol) by a variety of methods. One method used in medical nebulizers is to force the driving gas (propellant) through a small nozzle close to a supply of the liquid to be atomized. Droplets of the liquid are drawn into the stream of propellant by the Bernouilli effect where they may join a stream of low-pressure gas for delivery to the lungs or for humidification of the air in a room (fogging machine). The size of droplets may be reduced further if the stream of propellant and droplets impinges on an obstruction (anvil) or other spoiler.

The effect may be used for the humidification of anaesthetic gases, for environmental humidification or for atomizing local anaesthetic agents. The propellant may be provided from a high-pressure gas supply (e.g. aerosol can), or from a hand-squeezed bulb.

Audiometer n=4 c=2,3,4 r=3

Treatment for deafness can vary from the fitting of an electronic hearing aid to major surgery, depending on the origin of the problem. In almost every case an audiometer is used to discover the magnitude of the hearing loss and to assist in the diagnosis of the type of deafness. The commonest type of audiometer produces pure tones at set frequencies and known amplitudes through headphones worn by the patient who is required to indicate (by pressing a button) which of the tones he can hear. Variations exist which do not use headphones (free-field or bone conduction audiometers) and the tones may be replaced by words which the patient is required to recognize and repeat. A further category of audiometer exists, which does not require the co-operation of the patient, and can even be performed under general anaesthetic. These are electric response audiometers (ERA) which detect whether an auditory stimulus (tone or click) has been received at the cochlea (electrocochleograph – ECochG), the brain stem, the cortex (slow vertex response), or in auditory reflex arcs as may be detected from the electromyogram of the post auricular muscle (PAM), sometimes called the crossed acoustic response.

A very simple audiometer might have only a small number of tone frequencies, with rather large steps between the tone amplitude settings and may be for free field use only. Such a device would probably be used mainly outside the hospital for screening large numbers of people for hearing defects quickly (e.g. school children). Such audiometers may produce a warble tone instead of a steady tone to eliminate the problem of standing waves in the testing room. At the other end of the scale a single apparatus might be capable of producing the signals required (including masking noises) and recording the responses involved in several of the tests mentioned above.

Hearing testing in the hospital is performed almost exclusively in the audiology department where they also fit hearing aids and take the impressions necessary for the manufacture of ear moulds.

Tympanometry, by which the quality of sound transmission across the middle ear is assessed, is sometimes called middle ear audiometry, and thus the instrument used may be called an audiometer. However, in this case the principle of operation is completely different. An audible tone is fed into the ear but it is not important whether this is heard by the patient or not. For further details see Acoustic impedance bridge.

Auriscope n=50 c=1

Also known as an otoscope, the auriscope is a hand-held battery-powered light source and lens system for looking into the outer ear. Most have a detachable tip (speculum) which comes in a range of sizes. The bulb is usually energized via a rheostat (variable resistance) in order to control its brightness although this facility is normally used only in ophthalmic testing when the lens and speculum are detached and replaced by an ophthalmoscope attachment. Most auriscopes are monocular devices although binocular versions are available.

Auto analyser n=2 c=6,7 r=9

A large part of the work of the clinical chemistry laboratory in a hospital is to estimate the concentrations of various ions, molecules and enzymes in samples of body fluids taken from the tissues, blood, urine, cerebro-spinal fluid, etc. For many of these tests the analysis procedure consists of splitting the sample for the number of separate investigations requested, diluting these sub-samples, adding the reagents, heating, mixing, etc. and then analysing in a colorimeter, flame or spectrophotometer or other detector.

Since these tests are required in large numbers automated apparatus has become available which takes in samples at one end and prints the results at the other. There are three main types of auto analyser each with its own advantages and disadvantages.

1. Continuous flow analysers. These employ an intriguing system by which the subdivided sample and a quantity of reagent are drawn through a long narrow plastic tube to the detection device (colorimeter or flame photometer). The necessary chemical reaction takes place during the time the bolus of fluid is passing along the tube, and it may be accelerated by heating if this is necessary for the particular chemical process

involved. After a sample and quantity of reagent have been fed into the tube an air bubble is introduced followed by water, followed by another air bubble before the next sample. With this arrangement each sample with reagent is allowed to pass along the tube without mixing with any other in the same continuous flow stream. The meniscus of the bubble serves to clean the inside of the tube to prevent contamination of the samples. The Technicon SMA (sequential multiple analyser) series of auto analysers use continuous flow.

2. Centrifugal analysers. In these the sample and reagent are pipetted into wells (e.g. 30 of each) in the rotor of a centrifuge. When the centrifuge is started each sample and reagent pair is spun down into a cuvette on the edge of the rotor where they pass between the light source and photometer of a colorimeter. An electronic system identifies the photometric results to the correct sample and reagent cuvette, and can monitor the progress of the reaction in each cuvette. The end-point of each reaction can be identified and used in the same way as the continuous flow analyser, but it is also possible to identify reaction rate which is useful in estimating enzyme concentration. An example of a centrifugal analyser is the Centrifichem made by the Union Carbide Corporation (now marketed under the name Encore).

3. Discrete sample analyser. In these the sample is diluted and separated into a number of sub-samples appropriate to the number of tests requested. These are then mixed with reagents and the necessary time or heat treatment given before passing to a detector device to monitor the end point. Although this system appears more clumsy than the continuous flow analyser its advantage is that the machine can be programmed to perform only those tests which are requested, so saving on expense. Also it may be possible to have a bigger battery of tests available, though not all need to be performed on the same sample.

Autoclave n=6 c=3,4 r=2

Metal surgical instruments, and some rubbers and plastics may be sterilized by high-temperature steam. An autoclave is a sealed pressure vessel which exhausts the air and then admits steam under pressure (which can therefore be maintained at a temperature considerably above boiling point in atmospheric air). Since the air has been removed the steam will penetrate every part of the instruments being sterilized. Afterwards the chamber is evacuated again leaving the instruments dry.

Small autoclaves will operate from the electricity supply but larger types use the piped steam supplies. Instruments are often packed in special porous paper wrapping, sealed with an indicator tape, on which bands change colour when the sterilizing process is complete.

Auto-gamma counter n=3 c=5,6 r=3

This is an automated well counter for assessing the radioactive content of test samples. Several hundred samples may be moved along a conveyer and lowered one at a time into a scintillation counter of which the scintillation crystal is shaped into a well to receive the sample. The result of the counting from each sample is often handled by computer and the preparation of the samples is simpler than that required for a liquid scintillation counter. The crystal is housed in a thin aluminium can to exclude light but allow gamma rays to pass through. Gamma ray energies above about 20 keV may be counted.

Such devices may be found in the nuclear medicine, haematology, chemical pathology or immunology departments. A typical application would be the estimation of the amount of radioactive chromium in a blood sample.

Auto-transformer n=10 c=1,2

The mains supply voltage available at a wall socket in a hospital may not be appropriate for all equipment. This is most commonly encountered where American equipment requiring 110 V is to be used on the 250 V supply found in European hospitals. The solution to the problem is to use an auto-transformer which is a single coiled winding on a laminated iron core on which there are various tapping points to produce different voltages. The use of single winding means that the bulk of the device is much smaller than for a conventional double-wound transformer. Some auto-transformers can provide a variable output (a Variac) in which the number of turns of the coil presented in the output circuit can be varied by adjusting a control knob. Auto-transformers are most commonly encountered in the pathology departments where the equipment is drawn from a wide market. Often the suppliers of foreign equipment will incorporate an auto-transformer inside the equipment so that no additional device is required.

Averager n=5 c=4 r=3,9

Although this has a common meaning, in medical equipment it normally refers to an electrical signal averager of the type used for averaging the response to a stimulus (light, sound, or the use of a short-acting drug). The response being monitored may be the heart rate, EEG, EMG, blood pressure, etc. and these may undergo fluctuations due to external interference or natural variations. If the response evoked by the stimulus is likely to be small compared with these other fluctuations, signal averaging may be employed to demonstrate the effect of the stimulus alone. The usual method

23

is to repeat the test a number of times and add up all the responses so that natural fluctuations cancel out since they are not linked to the time of the stimulus. For evoked response averaging applied to an optical or auditory stimulus affecting the EEG the test may be repeated a large number of times in rapid succession so that a very small response may be detected in the presence of quite substantial noise. For a drug test, which may be carried out once only on each of a number of patients, the number of tests may be small.

Averagers are commonly found in the EEG, EMG and audiology clinics of hospitals and are usually microcomputers which hold the results in a computer memory so that each new result is added to the previous one in the computer memory. Tests performed using evoked response averagers include electric response audiometry (ERA), visual evoked response (VER), and electroretinogram (ERG).

Ayres T-piece c=1 r=2

A three-way connector for inclusion in the breathing circuit during anaesthesia. It has two wide-bore connectors which are in line and a narrow side arm for the fresh gas feed. It can be used in the T-piece circuit to provide non-rebreathing anaesthesia without the resistance to exhalation introduced by the usual expiratory valve.

B

B-scanner n=5 c=6 r=1

This is an ultrasonic device employing pulsed ultrasound in the megahertz (MHz) range which records the depth from which echoes arise and the position in an $X–Y$ plane. Depth into the body is usually displayed on the Y-axis of a CRT, distance along the skin surface in the direction of the scan is displayed on the X-axis and the echo amplitude is presented via the Z-modulation (brightness).

B-scanners were first used in the early 1960s for visualization of the foetus *in utero*, but have since been used for examining other organs within the body such as the heart, liver, kidneys, thyroid, bladder, spleen, and eyes.

Early B-scanners used a single transducer to send the ultrasound pulses and to detect the returning echoes. The transducer was moved over the skin manually so that the picture (a section) was built up over 10–15 seconds. Now the majority of ultrasonic scanners can produce a moving picture, either with a multi-element transducer which steers the ultrasound beam electronically, or the scanning motion is achieved using a rocking or rotating transducer or mirror.

B-scanners are found in X-ray departments and sometimes in ante-natal units. The main components are the transducer, a pulse generator, an echo amplifier, video drive circuits, beam steering and registration circuits and a display device, which may now include a computer type memory or scan converter to retain the image and allow some post-capture processing of the image.

Babywarmer n=5 c=3 r=4,6

Small babies cannot control the temperature of their own bodies very well. Premature babies are mostly nursed in incubators where the temperature of their environment can be closely controlled, and the temperature of the infant can also be monitored by a thermistor. Those at less thermal risk and those undergoing examination or treatment may be transferred to a babywarmer, which is a special cot having a large low-temperature radiant heater mounted above it. The energy radiated by the element may be controlled from a thermistor on the skin of the infant.

Back bar r=2

On a continuous flow anaesthetic machine the intermediate pressure (60 psi) gases from the cylinders or pipelines are fed into the low-pressure circuit at the flowmeter valves, where the flow rate of each gas is controlled and metered. The gases from the rotameters are mixed in a tube which runs across the back of the machine. This is the back bar, and it can have special fittings so that one or more vaporizers can be inserted, one at a time, into the flow of gas to introduce anaesthetic vapours. The downstream end of the back bar supplies the fresh gas outlet.

Bag squeezer r=2

This describes a type of automatic intermittent positive pressure ventilator which can be used in conjunction with a closed anaesthetic circuit. It relieves the anaesthetist of having to squeeze the breathing bag and provides more regular ventilation with controllable tidal volume and pressure, as well as the possibility of a negative pressure phase to draw air out of the lungs. The bag may be squeezed by a motor and levers, by a spring, or by adjustable weights. When driven by a motor (e.g. East Radcliffe ventilator) the ratio of the inspiratory and expiratory times may not be varied; however, where the bag is squeezed pneumatically by the 'bag in a bottle' principle (e.g. Blease pulmoflator) a whole range of timing options become available. If the bag is squeezed by a motor it is likely to be a constant volume generator. If, however, it is squeezed by a weight the result will be constant pressure with the volume limited by time or flow rate.

Ball float meter n=500 c=1 r=2

These are commonly used to monitor and set oxygen flow in oxygen therapy apparatus. They consist of a needle valve to control flow and a tapered tube containing a ball which is driven up the tube to a height depending on the flow of gas past it. The tube is triangular in internal section or trefoil. The mode of operation is similar to that of a rotameter but accuracy is less (typically 10% at 10 l/min). The scale engraved on the tube is read at the centre of the ball. The need for the tube to be exactly vertical is less than with a rotameter. They are usually connected to the gas source (pipeline connector or cylinder) with a connector which cannot be inserted into the wrong gas source. These are used in large numbers in hospital wards.

Ballistocardiograph n=0 c=5 r=9

Blood from the heart is mainly ejected upwards along the ascending aorta.

This produces a small downward accelerating force on the rest of the body, and this can be detected if the subject is laid on a special force platform. The forces involved are in the range 0–7 mg with frequency components from d.c. to 40 Hz. The platform requires a very low friction suspension and such devices have been used in research to develop techniques to assess the performance of the heart. They are not found in clinical use.

Barany box n=2 c=1

In audiometry, although sound may be presented to one ear it is by no means certain which ear picks up the sound, especially when there is a marked difference in the acuity of the ears. This problem is overcome by presenting a noise to the non-test ear, so making it temporarily deaf. Pure tone audiometers usually include a device for doing this (called a masker) but when tuning fork tests are undertaken, a Barany box is sometimes used. It is a very simple clockwork device which emits a rattling noise to the non-test ear. It is very crude and probably creates more problems than it solves since the noise is usually sufficient to impair the hearing of the ear being tested in addition to that of the non-test ear.

Basket anaesthetic machine n=0 r=2

This is an older type of anaesthetic machine on which gas cylinders are mounted in metal baskets and the pressure regulators are attached directly on to the cylinders. On modern machines the cylinders are each mounted on a yoke with a pin-index system to prevent connection of the wrong type of cylinder (i.e. the wrong gas).

Bed weighing system n=3 c=4

In dialysis, in intensive care, and in the treatment of patients suffering from burns a bed weighing system is useful for monitoring weight and weight changes. Patients suffering from fluid loss or undergoing fluid correction can be managed better if their weight can be monitored while they are in bed.

The instrument consists of four load cells which are placed under the wheels of the bed and a central control unit which calculates the total weight of the bed. Changes in total weight can then be monitored.

Bekesy Audiometer n=1 c=4 r=8

A semi-automatic pure tone audiometer may be used to eliminate the operator element in hearing testing. A Bekesy audiometer or Bekesy attachment for a conventional audiometer causes the tone to step automatically from one frequency to the next (or glide continuously through the frequency range), and the amplitude to increase and decrease, controlled by the patient pressing a button to indicate when he can hear the tones. The resulting audiogram is plotted automatically on an X–Y recorder. If the test is repeated using a bleeping rather than a continuous tone, further diagnostic information can be obtained from differences between the two results.

Belt respirator n=1 c=2 r=2

Alternating or intermittent pressures applied to the trunk may augment or replace the patient's own respiratory effort. This type of respirator consists of a flexible airtight bag wrapped around the chest which is repeatedly inflated by hand squeezing of a second bag, or is inflated by a machine. These can be useful if access to the airways is prevented by the procedure being undertaken. Belt respirators are sometimes called Pinkerton cuirass ventilators.

Beta counter n=2 c=5 r=3

The detection and measurement of radio-labelled compounds emitting gamma rays is usually achieved using a sodium iodide scintillation crystal in conjunction with a photomultiplier (PM) tube. At lower energies (below 20 keV) and with beta rays (up to 500 keV), the rays are excessively attenuated. This problem is overcome by mixing the scintillator with the sample in a light-tight vial in intimate contact with the PM tube. This is the principle of the beta counter, or liquid scintillation counter.

The scintillators are complex organic molecules, and secondary scintillators may be used to convert the wavelength to match the PM tube. The devices are intended for counting samples containing beta-emitting radionuclides such as tritium and carbon 14. They are found in hospital departments such as chemical pathology, nuclear medicine, and immunology.

Betatron n=1 c=5,6 r=4

High-energy X-rays (>25 MeV) can be produced by bombarding an X-ray target with an electron beam produced in a 'donut' shaped porcelain or glass circular tube between strong electromagnets. Control of the alternating magnetic flux (50–180 Hz) enables an electron beam to be steadily accelerated until released from the 'equilibrium orbit' by reducing the flux. The principle is somewhat similar to that used in the cyclotron. Such machines have been used in the radiotherapy department for the treatment of deep-seated tumours, although they are not often found in routine clinical use now.

Biofeedback apparatus n=1 c=3 r=4

This consists of a transducer, amplifier, signal processor and display. The object is to provide a visual or audible indication of some physiological function which it may be possible to learn to control. The signals monitored may include the ECG, EEG, EMG, plethysmogram, or thermal signal. Conditions to be controlled may include high blood pressure, consciousness, epilepsy, heart rate, insomnia, migraine, muscle spasm, or emotional stress.

Best known is the control of the EEG, particularly the alpha rhythm, as an aid to relaxation. In this case the alpha rhythm is extracted from the EEG and displayed as an optical or auditory signal, and the patient learns to increase or decrease the strength of the signal.

Bipolar coagulator

Surgical diathermy apparatus is used for cutting tissue without causing bleeding, and for arresting bleeding by heat coagulating the bleeding ends of small arterioles. A variation on this technique is bipolar diathermy in which high-frequency electric current is passed between the ends of a special forceps so that heating only occurs in a small region between the two arms of the device. This is more precise than monopolar diathermy and prevents the currents from passing through other parts of the body. Since the intention is to coagulate tissue and not to cut it, a diathermy set operating with a bipolar probe is sometimes called a bipolar coagulator. See also Surgical diathermy, and Bipolar surgical diathermy.

Bipolar surgical diathermy n=2 c=4 r=3,4

As an alternative to the conventional (monopolar) surgical diathermy, in which the electrical current flows from a small active probe through the body to a large indifferent electrode, the path of the current can be constrained to pass only through the tissue being treated. This is achieved using a special forceps in which the two halves of the instrument are insulated from one another and in effect one half becomes the source of the current and the other the destination, thus replacing the active and indifferent electrodes mentioned above.

Bipolar diathermy has the advantage that electric currents do not pass through parts of the body which are not being treated and also it is possible to be much more precise with the quantity of tissue being coagulated. For instance, a small blood vessel gripped between the jaws of the forceps will be coagulated, whereas tissue next to other parts of the forceps will not be heated at all. It is useful in microsurgery, but is often called for in other applications, particularly where there may be interference with the action of a cardiac pacemaker by the stray diathermy currents arising with monopolar systems.

Most modern diathermy machines can support the use of bipolar probes without modification. Older types are generally unsuitable since the indifferent connection to the machine is at earth potential, or is capacitively coupled to earth. An ideal bipolar diathermy current generator should be fully isolated from earth so that there will be no tendency for diathermy currents to circulate in the body to find other routes to earth. This is difficult to achieve at the frequencies used (1–3 MHz).

Bi-stable storage cathode ray tube (CRT) n=5 c=4

This allows a line image of a waveform or picture to be built up and retained on the face of a special cathode ray tube. Such devices are found in the electronics laboratory for examining the electrical signals found inside electronic apparatus, and they are also found in medical imaging apparatus such as in nuclear medicine and ultrasonic apparatus.

Lines drawn on the screen by the electron gun are retained as an electrostatic image on a mesh just behind the screen, and this can be retrieved by illuminating the mesh with a low-velocity electron beam from a flood gun. The phosphor layer on the CRT screen is activated in proportion to the electrostatic charge pattern retained on the mesh. New methods of retaining a stored image (such as digital storage mechanisms) are sought because it is difficult to obtain an image which has varying shades of brightness using the bi-stable CRT mechanism. This has particular disadvantages for ultrasonic B-scanners since the echo amplitude contains an important part of the information required for diagnosis. Bi-stable CRTs have been used for many years in ultrasound machines but have now been supplanted by newer techniques which can provide a true grey-scale image of the echo pattern.

Bladder stimulator n=1 c=2 r=6

This is a general term applied to electrical stimulators of the bladder or urethra. In some disorders of the urinary bladder normal emptying is impossible, usually due to disruption of the nerve supply. An electrical stimulator (usually implanted) can assist emptying of the bladder by stimulating the bladder muscle directly or by stimulating the nerves where they leave the spinal column. Only a small number of such devices have been implanted.

Stimulation of the urethra to assist closure in cases of urinary incontinence has been more successful and some hundreds of cases have been treated by implantable stimulators to provide enhanced contraction of the muscles in and around the urethra. The implants are usually passive and are energized by radio or inductive connection to a transmitter outside the body which the patient wears over the implant.

The main components of the system would be an external radio frequency pulse generator driving a coil applied to the skin over the implant. The implant usually consists of a receiving coil and a detector circuit feeding electrodes sewn into the muscles near the urethra.

Sometimes external stimulators are used to test the likely effect of an implanted stimulator or as a substitute for it. These may use electrodes mounted on a plug or pessary which fits into the rectum or vagina.

Blood flow meter n=5 c=3,4 r=3,9

Blood flow may need to be measured in three different situations. The rate of blood flow pumped by the heart (cardiac output) as a measure of heart performance, flow through arterial grafts at the time of surgery to check that the graft will perform satisfactorily, and flow in peripheral vessels may be measured to help in the diagnosis of the site and severity of vascular disease.

Cardiac output is usually measured using a dilution technique (thermal, dye, isotope), vascular graft performance is usually measured using an electromagnetic flow-meter and sometimes with an ultrasonic doppler flow-meter, and peripheral flow is usually assessed using an ultrasonic blood velocity or flow-meter. Peripheral flow is sometimes assessed using light, volume or impedance plethysmographs.

Further details may be found under the specific items mentioned above.

Blood gas analyser n=6 c=4,5 r=2,6,9

The partial pressures of oxygen and carbon dioxide in the blood are important indicators of the acid-base balance of the patient. Samples of arterial blood may be taken to the laboratory, but it is also common to have a blood gas analyser on hand in the intensive care unit, in the special care baby unit, and the labour ward. Modern analysers only require a very small sample of blood, but are relatively expensive and internally complex.

The partial pressure of oxygen (pO_2) measurement usually employs the Clark-type polarographic electrode in which oxygen diffuses through a membrane and is detected in a potassium chloride solution as the quantity of electric current generated between a glass-coated platinum electrode and a silver/silver chloride reference electrode. The necessary reactions occur under a polarizing voltage of 600–800 mV and the total current is limited by the very small exposed area on the platinum cathode (e.g. 20 μm diameter). The membrane is usually polypropylene although it can be Teflon.

Reactions in the Clark electrode are very sensitive to temperature and so exact control is necessary. The system is calibrated using two gases of known oxygen concentration. Measurement of carbon dioxide concentration is usually achieved in an assembly including two chambers, one for the specimen and a second containing a pH electrode bathed in a buffer solution of bicarbonate and sodium chloride. The two chambers are separated by a semipermeable membrane usually made of Teflon. This allows dissolved carbon dioxide to pass through but blocks the passage of charged particles. Carbon dioxide diffuses across the membrane to produce the same concentration in both chambers and the pH in the inner chamber increases or decreases respectively. The pH of the sample is measured by an inbuilt pH meter.

Blood gas estimations can also be performed non-invasively. Methods include infrared oximeters which typically fit on to the earlobe, or gas-sensitive membrane electrodes which may be fitted onto the skin (transcutaneous pO_2 and pCO_2 meters) or made as part of an intra-arterial probe. These latter types, though important, are still troublesome in use.

Blood leak detector r=3,9

In a haemodialysis machine there is always the possibility of rupture of the dialysing membrane with consequent leaking of blood into the dialysate. To identify this problem an optical blood leak detector is included to detect staining of the dialysate after it leaves the artificial kidney. This is normally an optical device which detects reduction in light transmission through the dialysate in a special cell which causes the machine to indicate that there is a fault, and also causes the machine to fail to a safe condition.

Blood leak detectors are normally an integral part of the haemodialysis machine, but may be a separate device on some machines. The chamber may be disposable on some modern machines.

Blood level detector r=3

During haemodialysis, blood passes from the patient through the artificial kidney (dialyser) and is returned to the body via a bubble trap. This is a broad chamber in which bubbles rise, thus preventing air being pumped back into the patient via the venous return tube which leaves the chamber at the bottom. As the quantity of air at the top of the trap builds up, so the blood level falls.

A blood level detector may be a photoelectric detector on the trap to show when blood has fallen below an acceptable level. The technique is not completely foolproof because of frothing, and so a second photoelectric detector on the narrow outlet tube is sometimes used. If air is detected, or the blood level falls too low, an alarm sounds and the dialysis may be interrupted until the condition is corrected. On some modern machines air may be detected in the blood by an ultrasonic detector combined with a clamp for extra safety.

The blood level detector may be an integral part of the dialysis machine, or it may be a separate device.

Blood loss meter n=2 c=4 r=2

A knowledge of the amount of blood lost during surgery is valuable for the management of the patient. Blood lost includes that carried away on swabs, on the drapes, gowns, and on the floor. There may also be loss into the suction apparatus and some blood is immobilized within the patient. There is no perfect way to assess all the losses but a practical method of estimating losses into swabs and drapes does exist.

This device, sometimes called a perometer, looks like a small washing machine and agitates the drapes and swabs in a haemolysing solution. The concentration of blood in the solution is then estimated by a colorimetric method (to estimate the quantity of haemoglobin present), or the electrical impedance is measured to estimate blood electrolytes.

Both these methods are tedious to perform and are not often used.

Blood pressure monitor/meter r=6,9

This may monitor blood pressure in the chambers of the heart, in arteries, veins, or in the capillary bed. The most common pressure to be measured is the arterial pressure, and this can be obtained indirectly (from outside the body), or measured directly through catheters or needles placed within the blood stream.

Indirect blood pressure monitors include the common sphygmomano-meter which records the external pressure required to occlude an artery within a limb. Since the arterial blood pressure is pulsatile it is possible to identify the point at which the blood pressure is just able to open the artery (systolic, or peak blood pressure) and the blood pressure at which the artery just closes momentarily at its lowest internal pressure (diastolic blood pressure). These two points may be detected by listening through a stethoscope placed on the skin downstream of the pressure cuff, or it may be detected automatically from the pulse waveform produced in the pressure cuff, by the sounds detected by a microphone on the skin under the pressure cuff, or by an ultrasonic doppler transducer which detects the arterial wall movement. Double cuff methods are used in the oscillometer and haemo-tonometer. Automated indirect blood pressure recorders are sometimes incorporated into other instruments monitoring temperature, respiration rate, and heart rate.

33

To record the waveform of the arterial pressure a catheter or needle must be introduced into the artery and connected to an electrical pressure transducer. Such devices must record the waveform faithfully and this requires a frequency response of at least ten times the heart rate (e.g. 15 Hz). Good frequency response is particularly important when recording within the chambers of the heart in the cardiac catheter laboratory and the fidelity of the recording depends on the diameter, length, and compliance of the catheter, and on the exclusion of all air from the system.

Blood pump n=20 c=2,3 r=3

The pumping of blood is required during haemodialysis and during open heart surgery. Roller pumps, which produce a peristaltic flow of blood, are the most common. These have the advantage that the pump mechanism does not come into contact with blood. The mode of operation is for a soft tube carrying the blood to be pressed into a special groove (shoe) and two or more rollers on a rotating spindle occlude the tube in turn pushing the blood forward. The design of the shoe and the rollers must be such that the tube is always occluded at at least one point to prevent leakback.

In haemodialysis the pump may be incorporated into the machine or may be a separate device which controls the flow of blood from the body and drives it through the dialyser.

Blood damage (haemolysis) is reduced if the following precautions are taken:

1. The tubing compressed by the rollers should be relatively soft but not too soft. Very soft tubing allows considerable movement between the tube walls and the roller.
2. Use the largest diameter of tube possible.
3. If the rollers are set so that they only just occlude the tube this reduces haemolysis and tube wear.
4. Use lubricants (e.g. silicone jelly).

Blood velocity meter n=5 c=4 r=3

A continuous ultrasonic wave in the megahertz region is scattered as it passes through blood. The back-scattered part of the signal can be collected by a receiving transducer next to the transducer emitting the continuous waves, and the returning signal will be shifted in frequency in proportion to the velocity of the blood in the vessel. This doppler frequency shift can be detected and applied to a frequency meter (e.g. zero crossing detector) or frequency analyser to produce a signal proportional to blood velocity. The doppler frequency shift will normally fall inside the audible frequency range for the practical range of ultrasonic frequencies and blood velocities.

Unfortunately blood within a vessel is not all travelling at the same velocity. Blood at the centre may be moving at a different rate and even in a different direction from the blood near the vessel walls. To overcome this problem the velocity may be sampled at several points across the vessel and the average velocity computed, although in other cases the shape of the flow profile is sufficient information for the diagnosis required. Alternatively a more crude average of velocity may be discovered using a frequency meter, usually counting the number of zero crossings occurring each second. A major improvement in accuracy may be achieved by resolving the forward and reverse flow separately by identifying those doppler shifted components which lie above the transmitted frequency (flow towards the transducer) from those below.

A useful assessment of blood flow in peripheral vessels can be made using the most simple form of ultrasonic device and listening to the doppler signals through headphones. As the pitch rises the blood is flowing faster, as it would at a constriction in the vessel. This type of device uses a probe containing both transmitting and receiving transducer elements which is placed on the skin lubricated by a drop of coupling jelly. The instrument contains an oscillator to generate the ultrasonic frequency (typically 10 MHz), a receiving amplifier, a simple envelope or synchronous detector, and an audio amplifier. If forward and reverse flow can be separated the two signals are presented to the left and right ear separately.

More complex devices provide metered or chart records of the flow. The actual flow waveforms may be recognized as indicating different disorders such as constriction in the larger vessels or high impedance to flow in the extremities.

Blood warmer $n=20$ $c=2$

During blood transfusion it is desirable to pre-heat the blood to the body temperature. The most common device for this is a temperature-controlled water bath into which a coil of tubing is immersed through which the blood flows. The temperature of the bath is normally maintained slightly above body temperature to allow for any cooling in the feed tube to the patient. The device consists of a bath with a heating element, a stirrer (usually) to ensure even distribution of temperature, and electronic circuitry to control the temperature and to provide an over-temperature limit in the event of system failure or low water level.

Alternative devices exist in which the blood is passed through a coil or bag enclosed between dry heating plates. These types have similar control and alarm circuits. Blood warmers are also known as haemoheaters.

Blow-off valve r=2

This is a pressure relief valve intended to prevent the build-up of pressure beyond safe limits. It normally consists of a plunger and a spring of adjustable tension. Such valves are found in anaesthetic equipment and, incidentally, in any steam pressure apparatus (e.g. autoclaves). An example of the use of a pressure relief valve in an anaesthetic circuit would be to limit the pressure which can be applied to the patient's lungs by an anaesthetic machine to (say) 60 cmH$_2$O. Sometimes blow-off valves are used as pressure regulators by allowing them to vent surplus gases, thereby retaining the circuit pressure at the blow-off pressure.

Bodok seals r=2

Where a pin-indexed valve block on a medical gas cylinder is connected to a machine (e.g. anaesthetic machine valve yoke) the block is pressed on to a washer of non-combustible material to form the high-pressure seal between the two. Before medical gas cylinders are fitted it is important that the state of this seal be examined and a replacement fitted if there are signs of damage. Bodok (sometimes called a Dowty seal) is really a proprietary name but it is generally applied to these types of washer.

Body box n=1 c=4,5 r=3,9

A whole body plethysmograph may be used to estimate the residual volume of the lungs and make measurements of other variables of interest in the study of lung function. The main element in a whole body plethysmograph is the body box, which is a sealed chamber, rather like a telephone box, in which the patient sits and breathes through a tube passing out of the box. Since the volume of the patient will change during the breathing cycle, so the air pressure inside the box will vary in sympathy. The residual volume within the lungs can be found by measuring the pressure in the airway when the patient tries to inhale from a closed tube. The residual volume can then be calculated from the increased volume of the lungs and the reduced pressure during attempted inspiration. The body box will be found in a lung function laboratory.

Body respirator n=0 c=4 r=2

This is a device for augmenting or replacing the spontaneous respiratory effort of the patient, and is used in intensive care, or at the patient's home. This type works by applying alternating force or pressure to the outside of the chest and may include the whole body cabinet type (iron lung), cuirass, and belt (Pinkerton cuirass) types.

Bone conduction transducer/receiver r=8

Also known as a bone vibrator, this is an electromagnetic transducer which is normally positioned behind the ear on the mastoid bone and kept in position by a sprung headband. When fed with audio frequency signals it imparts a corresponding vibration to the skull and thence to both inner ears. It has two principal applications:

1. As an output device for an audiometer used in audiology departments. This can be used for testing patients' hearing as an adjunct to testing with conventional earphones (known as air conduction). Comparison of the results thus achieved enables the clinician to distinguish whether a hearing loss is attributable to the external or middle ear (a conductive loss) or inner ear (sensory loss).
2. Some patients who wear a hearing aid cannot wear an ear mould which is the normal mechanism for coupling the hearing aid to the patient's ear. Instead its output is routed via a bone vibrator. The main disadvantage of this transducer is its very high distortion, its limited output, and its relative discomfort and obtrusiveness.

Bone saw n=6 c=4

Hand saws looking very like carpenters' saws are sometimes used for working on large bones. However, there are power saws available which fall into electric and pneumatic types. The electric types usually have a blade which vibrates. The advantage of having a vibrating rather than a rotating blade is that, if the vibrations are small, cutting will only occur in hard materials (e.g. bone) but will not occur in soft materials. Compressed air powered saws are more common particularly for orthopaedic surgery. They often come as a kit consisting of an air-operated motor and foot-operated speed control, and a set of fittings for sawing, drilling, screwing and pinning. They are intended to work from nitrogen or air at 7 bar pressure which may be provided by pipeline or from cylinders.

Since the surgeon normally holds the motor during the sawing operation the whole device must be sterilizable. Pneumatic types are more amenable to total sterilization.

Bone vibrator r=8

Also known as bone conduction transducer or bone conduction receiver, this is an electromagnetic transducer which is normally positioned behind the ear on the mastoid bone and kept in position by a sprung headband. When fed with audio frequency signals it imparts a corresponding vibration to the skull and thence to both inner ears. It has two principal applications:

1. As an output device for an audiometer used in audiology departments. This can be used for testing patients' hearing as an adjunct to testing with conventional earphones (known as air conduction). Comparison of the results thus achieved enables the clinician to distinguish whether a hearing loss is attributable to the external or middle ear (a conductive loss) or inner ear (sensory loss).

2. Some patients who wear a hearing aid cannot wear an ear mould, which is the normal mechanism for coupling the hearing aid to the patient's ear. Instead its output is routed via a bone vibrator. The main disadvantage of this transducer is its very high distortion, its limited output, and its relative discomfort and obtrusiveness.

Bosun oxygen failure warning device r=2

The name originates from the Bosun's whistle, since it blows a whistle when the oxygen supply to an anaesthetic machine fails. Loss of oxygen supply is very serious since if no warning is given the patient may be breathing 100% nitrous oxide. If this situation continues for a few minutes the patient may be seriously injured or killed. Various designs of warning device are available, some of which automatically interrupt the supply of other gases. However, this type simply whistles for a few seconds and brings a light on. The whistle is operated by oxygen contained in a small bellows which empties when the inlet pressure falls. Disadvantages of this type of alarm are that the nitrous oxide supply must be present and the battery and bulb must be maintained.

Bourdon gauge (manometer) n=300 c=1 r=2

This is an elaboration of the aneroid manometer used for higher pressures (up to 2000 psi). The corrugated cylinder of the aneroid manometer is replaced by a curved or spiral flattened tube which attempts to straighten when pressure is applied to the inside of it. The free end of the tube is connected to a rack and pinion to which a pointer is attached. These types of gauge are found on gas cylinders to indicate the pressure of the contents (and by inference the fullness). They are also found on anaesthetic apparatus to show the pressure of the pipelines (4 bar, 60 psi in UK). Where they are used on cylinders which contain liquids (e.g. compressed carbon dioxide, nitrous oxide, cyclopropane) the pressure is not a good guide to the fullness since pressure only falls significantly when all the liquid has been evaporated.

Boyles bottle (vaporizer) n=30 c=1 r=2

The Boyles vaporizer and similar types of 'bottle' are used on anaesthetic machines to vaporize ether, VAM, penthrane, trilene, etc. There is no calibration and no form of temperature compensation. It fits on to the back bar of an anaesthetic machine (i.e. downstream of the flowmeters) and has a lever to cause the gas flow to pass through, or to bypass the 'bottle'. Concentration of vapour is changed by depressing or withdrawing a plunger which causes the gases to come into more or less intimate contact with the liquid. The bottle containing the agent can be unscrewed and replaced by another.

Quite a number of these units are still seen in hospitals but they are not often used.

Boyles machine n=40 c=4 r=2

This is a trade name for a type of anaesthetic machine which is named after its inventor (an anaesthetist). However, the term is in common use to describe any general-purpose continuous flow anaesthetic machine intended to provide a variable mixture of gases and vapours for general anaesthesia. Modern machines are really quite unlike the original 1917 device.

Brachial stethoscope c=1 r=2

During anaesthesia, indirect blood pressure measurement may be performed by the anaesthetist using a brachial stethoscope. This is simply a strap-on stethoscope head with a long tube attaching it to the ear-pieces. It fits under a cuff encircling the patient's arm which can be inflated and deflated remotely so that the drapes do not have to be disturbed.

Breast pump n=3 c=2

Breast milk may be drawn off for feeding by bottle using a suction device and reservoir employing a suction cup about 6 cm in diameter which fits over the end of the breast. Hand-operated types are available with a simple piston action, and there are also electrically operated versions. More complex types provide a pulsating suction for simulated natural feeding.

Breathing circuit r=2

The breathing circuit or breathing system is that part of an anaesthetic apparatus which is downstream of the back bar. It includes reservoir and rebreathing bags, the corrugated flexible hoses, absorbers, facepiece, and some ventilator components. Pressure in the breathing circuit is always close to atmospheric pressure, except for the small pressure required for positive pressure ventilation.

There are two main types of breathing circuit:

1. Rebreathing (closed circuits), in which part or all of the expired gases are intentionally re-inspired.
2. Non-rebreathing circuits in which new gases are supplied for each breath, and any rebreathing which occurs is due to dead space in the breathing circuit.

Breathing machine n=70 c=1,4 r=2

This is another name for a ventilator intended to provide assisted breathing. The term covers such types as:

1. Resuscitators, which are usually portable.
2. Body respirators, which assist breathing by applying pressure to the outside of the chest.
3. Lung ventilators, which apply intermittent positive pressure to the inside of the lungs (usually through an endotracheal tube).
4. Rocking apparatus, which assists breathing by making the weight of abdominal contents move the diaphragm.

Breathing tube/hose n=500 c=1 r=2

This is the 'elephant tube' used to connect between components of the breathing circuit on anaesthetic apparatus. Its usual form is black antistatic corrugated tube with push fit/twist or lockable terminations (one male and one female) to fit other components of the breathing circuit. They need to be wide bore to present minimal resistance to breathing and the corrugations prevent kinking. The tubing sections usually hang down between the facepiece and absorber, etc. and this is said to reduce infection of the apparatus by trapping moisture at the bottom of the drape.

Bronchoscope n=10 c=2,3,4 r=2,4

This is a telescope for examining the larger airways in the lungs in the anaesthetized patient. Traditionally these have been straight tubes about 8 mm in diameter with a small electric light bulb near the end, and powered by a battery. The bronchoscope may also fit down the centre of a special cuffed endotracheal tube so that the lungs may be inflated for ease of viewing or for artificial ventilation.

Since the introduction of flexible (fibre-optic) endoscopes, new possibilities have arisen, including viewing further into the lungs. Instruments can be passed through small channels in the endoscope for excising tissue for sampling (biopsy) or for treatment. In common with other flexible endoscopes illumination is provided from a high-intensity light source through a fibre-optic bundle and the image is focused on to the end of a coherent bundle which conveys the focused light point for point to a viewing eyepiece. To achieve an image definition of 200 points by 200 points 40 000 fibres are required to be laid in exact symmetry along the length of the scope.

A bronchoscope would normally be passed during general anaesthesia.

Bubble oxygenator r=4

This is used to replace the function of the lung during heart surgery. The venous blood is passed up a vertical column through which bubbles of oxygen are rising. Oxygen enters the blood and carbon dioxide is released. The column may be a number of vertical tubes or a bag in which a fine mesh acts as a spoiler to promote mixing of the gas and blood. At the top of the column, the gases and blood form a foam from which the bubbles coalesce and are removed. On exit from the column blood passes through a filter and a bubble trap. The oxygenator may also include a cooling device to lower the body temperature of the patient to extend the time available for surgery. Reheating of the blood is often required during the latter stages of the procedure.

Bubble oxygenators are included in the heart–lung machine for cardiac surgery.

Membrane oxygenators also exist in which the gases and blood are separated by a semipermeable membrane.

Bubble trap r=3,9

When blood must be drawn from the body and then returned to it, bubbles of air may develop due to leaks, pressure changes in the circuit, or arising from the oxygenation process in a heart–lung machine.

The purpose of a bubble trap is to allow these bubbles to rise in a special chamber from which the blood leaves at the bottom. In haemodialysis special alarm circuitry is linked either to a blood level detector to identify when the air removed from the circuit displaces the blood downwards below an acceptable level, or there may be an optical or ultrasonic detector to show when bubbles are passing back to the patient.

The bubble trap is normally part of the disposable tubing set used for the procedure.

Bucky diaphragm r=7

The term 'Bucky' arises from the Potter-Bucky diaphragm, which was the first moving secondary radiation grid for X-ray sets. It is an assembly which is usually located under the table of a diagnostic X-ray set and holds the

X-ray film cassette and the secondary radiation grid. The grid is used to prevent secondary X-ray emission from the patient reaching the X-ray film, and is formed from a large number of thin strips of lead separated by a radiolucent material. To prevent the outline of the grid from appearing on the film a mechanism is provided for moving the grid during exposure. The Bucky is mounted on bearings which permit movement along rails under the X-ray table so that the grid and film can be moved to an appropriate position under the patient. The Bucky is used with most diagnostic X-ray equipment.

Although it is usually found as an integral part of the X-ray set, it may also be a separate device which can be used vertically or with an ordinary hospital trolley. For ward and theatre work, and with rapid X-ray film changers stationary grids are often used.

Bull-nosed cylinder valves r=2

This type of valve is used on medical gas cylinders which do not have the pin-index safety system. The turn-off mechanism points to one side and the gases are delivered vertically. They are commonly used for supplying gas for oxygen therapy (in conjunction with a reducing valve and flowmeter), and on emergency trolleys. One can also find 'hand wheel' cylinders on which there is a knob on the top of the cylinder valve and the gas comes out to the side. These systems are seen more often on larger cylinders such as those used for powering air-driven tools in operating theatres, etc.

C

C-scanner (ultrasonic) n=0 c=6 r=1

This is an ultrasonic scanning device which builds an image of a plane in the tissue which is perpendicular to the ultrasonic beam. This was originally done by time gating the returning echoes to correspond only to the chosen depth into the tissue. However, modern computerized tomography makes reconstruction of any plane of the tissue feasible.

C-scanning, though theoretically useful, has not gained wide acceptance in clinical ultrasound practice.

Cabinet ventilator n=0 c=4 r=2

Breathing can be assisted by placing the patient in a box with an airtight seal around the neck, leaving only the head outside. If air is pumped in and out of the box to create alternating high and low pressure, the chest will rise and fall ensuring ventilation of the lungs. This is the machine known to the public as the artificial lung or iron lung used in the management of polio. It is rarely used today because intermittent positive pressure ventilation, involving direct internal inflation and deflation of the lungs, is so much more effective and convenient for most requirements.

Calipers (ultrasonic) r=1

Although this term has an obvious meaning, it arises in medical instrumentation as part of an A- or B-scanner. One use of ultrasonic examination of the body is to measure the size of organs or tumours, and this requires a special facility to measure distances between points on the image.

On the A-scan, calipers usually take the form of bright dots on the A-scan line which can be adjusted in position to mark the two echoes representing the boundaries of the organ in question. This technique has been used extensively in obstetrics to measure the bi-parietal diameter (BPD) of the foetal head to estimate the age of the foetus. It can provide very accurate measurement of distance but it is not suitable where the two points required do not lie on a straight line from the skin surface into the body.

On B-scans, calipers are presented as bright dots, crosses, or a circle, which can be moved by a 'joy-stick' control to mark any two points on the screen. An electronic circuit calculates and displays the distance between these two points. An extension of this method is to draw a complete plan of the boundary of an organ or lesion with a joy-stick or light pen and have the internal computer calculate the circumference or area contained within the boundary.

Caloric apparatus n=1 c=3,4

Patients with problems of vertigo or dizziness are often referred for vestibulometric tests. One of the most common tests is called the caloric test in which the patient's ear canal is heated or cooled by the introduction of warm or cool water (the usual temperatures are 44 and 30°C, although more extreme temperatures are applied when air is used rather than water).

This has the effect of heating or cooling the temporal bone and thus the semi-circular canals of the human balance mechanism, causing eddy currents in the fluid within the canals. These eddy currents cause the patient to experience a feeling of motion, resulting in eye movements called jerk nystagmus. The speed or duration of this nystagmus can be measured subjectively by using an infrared viewer or Frenzel glasses, or objectively using an electronystagmograph. These measurements are a crude indication of the sensitivity of the balance mechanism under test.

The caloric apparatus is the thermostatically controlled water tanks which comprise an earthed metal tank, circulating pump, dial thermometer and heating element with thermostatic control.

Calorimeter

This is a device for measuring the quantity of heat released by a chemical or physical reaction. They are used in chemistry to determine heat of reaction, and in medical work to determine the quantity of ultrasonic radiation delivered by a particular ultrasonic therapy or diagnostic set.

In this ultrasonic example it takes the form of an insulated box containing a fluid which absorbs ultrasonic energy and converts it into heat. The internal structure of the box provides a multiple reflection path for the ultrasonic beam so that it passes many times through the absorbing medium (usually an oil) until the energy is fully absorbed. The ultrasonic transducer is applied to a thin plastic or glass window into the chamber and the device is calibrated by an electric heater and stirrer to compare the heat generated by the ultrasonic beam over a period of a few minutes to that generated by a known quantity of electrical energy. Such devices would normally be found in the medical physics department.

Capnometer/capnograph n=2 c=4

This measures carbon dioxide concentration in expired gases. It is used during anaesthesia and intensive care, and in lung function studies. In intensive care it may be used as a substitute for blood gas determinations or to monitor the performance of assisted ventilation.

The commonest type of capnometer uses changes in the infrared light transmission properties in gas mixtures containing carbon dioxide (see Infrared gas analyser). Since the concentration of oxygen, nitrous oxide, and carbon monoxide interferes with the transmission of infrared in mixtures containing carbon dioxide, corrections must be made if these are present. In some devices rapid responses are possible to allow detection of breath by breath carbon dioxide variation, and indication of the concentration occurring at the end of expiration.

A typical instrument contains the infrared transducer, a small pump to draw the gases through a narrow tube connected to the breathing circuit, a water trap, controls and a display unit. A pen recorder is sometimes added which can produce a plot of carbon dioxide percentage throughout the breathing cycle. The instrument may be combined with an oxygen analyser for some applications.

Carbon dioxide absorber n=20 c=2 r=2

This can apply to any material or device for absorbing carbon dioxide but it usually refers to a device for inclusion in a rebreathing anaesthetic circuit. The expired gases pass through it and are then re-inspired together with a small supplement of fresh anaesthetic gases.

The absorber may be a canister in line with the connection from the breathing bag to the patient or it may be a canister with appropriate valves for inclusion in a circle system. The carbon dioxide is absorbed in soda-lime (calcium hydroxide plus additives) or another mixture with similar properties. The lime is supplied as granules or pellets, often with a colour indicator to show when it is spent and needs changing.

Carbon dioxide analyser n=2 c=4

Measurement of carbon dioxide in expired gases is important in lung function studies, and in intensive care where the expired carbon dioxide level may be used as a substitute for blood gas analysis, or to reduce the frequency at which blood sampling is required. The commonest method of carbon dioxide determination is by measuring the absorption of infrared light passing through the gas mixture. Sampling types exist, often using a Golay cell, but on-line (real time) analysers also exist which can produce graphical representation of the carbon dioxide variation during breathing or assisted ventilation.

The method is fast acting and accurate except for interference by the presence of other gases (e.g. carbon monoxide) and the accuracy is modified by the presence of different oxygen and nitrous oxide concentrations. These latter are often compensated for by setting controls on the main instrument. However, to make the necessary adjustments, some knowledge of the approximate levels of oxygen and nitrous oxide is required. See also Capnometer, and Infrared gas analyser.

Slower acting, and more accurate versions exist which include a moisture absorber.

Carbon dioxide cystometer n=1 c=4

A cystometer is a device for recording the changes in bladder pressure as filling occurs. Although this can be performed as the bladder fills naturally, it is normal to test the bladder response to filling at medium or rapid filling rates (e.g. 30 ml/min or 100 ml/min). Most cystometry is performed using water or saline as the filling medium through a urethral catheter, the pressure being measured through this same catheter or a separate channel within the same catheter, or through a suprapubic puncture needle. Such devices are used widely for the investigation of causes of urinary incontinence and retention.

A variation on this theme is to use carbon dioxide as the filling medium. This allows a relatively dry procedure which need not be performed in hospital and the responses of the bladder are claimed to be similar to those found with water or saline. The normal cystometrogram shows a sustained low pressure throughout filling (e.g. 10–15 cmH$_2$O). However, in many cases there are involuntary contractions of the bladder during the filling process indicating an unstable or irritable bladder, a condition which is relatively difficult to treat.

Carbon dioxide insufflation apparatus n=5 c=3,4

This delivers carbon dioxide under low pressure to open up a space within the body. The most common application is to give a sufficiently large viewing area during endoscopy. An example is in laparoscopy when the viewing instrument is passed through a small incision in the abdomen. A space is created by carbon dioxide insufflation for viewing and internal surgery. Insufflation has also been used in the uterus as a diagnostic and treatment method to pass the gas up the length of the fallopian tubes.

Carbon dioxide is used since it will be readily absorbed into the tissues after the procedure, and also it will suppress combustion of flammable gases during surgical diathermy (e.g. in the bowel). The apparatus normally consists of a carbon dioxide cylinder, a regulator to reduce the pressure, and a small rotameter flowmeter and needle valve to control the rate of flow. Sometimes a pressure gauge and relief valve are included. Such devices are commonly found in operating theatres.

Carbon monoxide analyser n=1 c=4 r=3

This is an infrared gas analyser similar to that used for carbon dioxide estimations but responding to absorption at a different characteristic wavelength. They are used in transfer factor analysis to determine the rate of transfer of oxygen from the air to the blood. The determination cannot be achieved directly with oxygen since there is simultaneous transfer to and from the blood.

Carbon monoxide is used in small concentrations since it is readily absorbed and not immediately released. Such devices are used in the lung function laboratory.

Cardiac angiography apparatus n=1 c=7 r=4

This is a system used in a cardiac catheter laboratory to visualize the passage of blood through the chambers of the heart and the great vessels. A bolus of X-ray opaque contrast medium is injected from a high-pressure pump through a catheter placed at the starting point for the investigations. It may be injected into the coronary artery to demonstrate the location and severity of plaque build-up. It may be injected just downstream of a heart valve to give an indication of the amount of regurgitation through the valve or it may be injected through a distant vessel. Planimetric measurement of the chambers of the heart as seen on the video screen may provide information on the size of the heart chambers and the ejection fraction. This procedure may be performed at the same time as pressure measurements in the chambers of the heart and great vessels to investigate the performance of valves or to demonstrate septal defects.

Apart from the high-pressure pump, the apparatus is an X-ray machine with a fluoroscopic screen, coupled to a video system. It may also have a cine, or rapid film changing capability and may allow visualization in two planes at once.

Cardiac catheterization equipment n=1 c=7,8 r=9

Cardiac catheterization combines several techniques to assess haemodynamic function and cardiovascular structure. Cardiac catheterization is performed in almost all patients in whom heart surgery is contemplated. The procedure is performed in a specialized laboratory equipped with X-ray systems for visualizing heart structures and a battery of supplementary equipment for recording cardiac output, measuring respiratory and blood gases, blood oxygen saturation, and metabolic products. The injection of X-ray contrast medium into the ventricles or aorta allows assessment of ventricular or aortic function, and injection into the coronary arteries makes possible the assessment of coronary artery disease. A catheter may be passed from a peripheral vessel up into all four chambers of the heart to identify and recognize the characteristic pressure waveforms. By multichannel pressure recording the pressure gradients across all four valves can be measured.

Balloon-tipped flow-directed catheters may be used to make these recordings without the need for fluoroscopy and also the balloon may be passed into the pulmonary artery to record the wedge pressure when it becomes jammed in the pulmonary circulation. Blood samples may be drawn from within the various chambers and vessels and these may be used to determine blood gas partial pressure and metabolic products such as lactate, pyruvate, carbon dioxide, or the concentration of substances which have been injected such as radioactive materials or coloured dyes.

Cardiac output may be determined by the Fick method, dye dilution, thermal dilution or impedance cardiography.

Cardiac microphone r=9

Some information about the functioning of the heart may be obtained using a simple stethoscope, listening to the heart sounds. These sounds correspond to the opening and closing times of the main valves but there are others which are not always perceptible. A much more comprehensive analysis of the heart sounds can be made using a phonocardiograph by which the heart sounds are presented as their original or modified waveforms on a high speed chart recorder. The microphone for this is usually a crystal microphone set back from the skin in a noise-excluding housing, although contact types are also used. Normal heart sounds and murmurs occur in the frequency range 25–2000 Hz. Background noise and patient movement may create serious problems during phonocardiography. This may be overcome in the cardiac catheterization procedure by recording sounds from within the heart using a phonocatheter, or if miniature pressure transducers are mounted on the catheter, to record pressures within the chambers of the heart. These transducers may have sufficient frequency response to record the heart sounds as well.

Cardiac output computer n=3 c=4 r=3,9

The rate at which the heart pumps blood can be calculated from the concentration which a known quantity of an inert indicator reaches when injected into the blood stream close to the heart. The concentration of a dye (usually indocyanine green – ICG) can be detected in the pulmonary artery (i.e. leaving the heart) when it has been injected through a catheter opening into the right atrium. The concentration rises and then falls, and the cardiac output is calculated by computer from this curve using information about the quantity of dye injected and the calibration constant of the densitometer. This is an invasive procedure since the catheter must be fed up to the heart through an artery, usually the brachial artery. The correct position of the injection catheter eye and the collecting eye may be identified using X-ray screening (during cardiac catheterization) or by monitoring the pressure waveform at each point through the catheter itself.

An alternative to using a dye is to inject a bolus of cold saline and calculate the cardiac output from the dip in temperature sensed in the pulmonary artery. The temperature profile will follow the same course as the dye concentration. Thermal dilution has the advantage that the procedure may be repeated many times without loading the blood with toxic material, and is therefore sometimes applied in the intensive care unit.

The apparatus consists of an injection pump (usually), a special catheter which may be expensive and intended for single use only, and the computer itself.

Another method of calculating cardiac output during cardiac catheterization which does not involve an injection is the Fick method. In this case the indicator is oxygen. Consumption is measured by a spirometer in which exhaled carbon dioxide is absorbed to allow calculation of the quantity of oxygen used (a typical figure is 0.25 l/min). Samples of blood are taken through catheters, one in an artery of the arm or leg, and another in the pulmonary artery. The flow rate is then calculated from the formula:

$$F = (dm/dt) / (C_a - C_v)$$

where F is the blood flow in litres/minute, dm/dt is the consumption of oxygen in litres/minute, C_a is the arterial concentration of oxygen in litres/litre, and C_v is the venous concentration of oxygen in litres/litre.

Blood oxygen concentration is normally calculated by an optical method (see Oximeter).

There is also a method of calculating cardiac output using electrical impedance measurements on the chest but this has not been widely accepted.

Cardiac pacemaker n=50 c=3 r=3,4,6

The muscles of the heart must contract in the correct sequence to allow adequate times for filling and pumping. The timing mechanism depends upon the correct action of a natural pacemaker in the heart and the correct delays and distribution of the signal in the muscle and nerves of the heart. There are a number of congenital or acquired conditions in which the triggering (pacing) and timing mechanisms are disrupted, and for which a cardiac pacemaker may be a part of the treatment.

The pacemaker is an electrical stimulator with electrodes usually applied directly to the heart and providing pulses of a fixed rate (asynchronous pacemaker) or it may provide pulses only when the natural pulse fails to appear (demand pacemaker). There are many sub-classifications of cardiac pacemakers and these are mentioned briefly in the entry under Pacemaker.

Cardiff infusion system n=1 c=4

Drugs which cause the uterus to contract are commonly used to induce labour. These drugs are normally fed into a vein using a metered or pumped infusion system.

The Cardiff infusion system provides a complete control loop to regulate the flow of the drug according to the strength of the resulting uterine contractions. The infusion system may operate through connections to a cardiotocograph to derive the contraction signals, or may contain both measuring and control circuitry in the same housing.

Such systems are not often used, partly because of the unreliability of the uterine contraction signal. If the contractions are not recorded properly the device may demand an increase in the rate of infusion when none is required.

Cardiff swivel r=2

This is a terminal device for the fresh gas outlet on the front of some anaesthetic machines. It has a standard 22 mm taper (15 mm for paediatric use) to take a T-piece connecting to the breathing bag and patient circuit, and the whole device can be swivelled to deliver in the most convenient direction.

Cardiopulmonary bypass apparatus n=2 c=5,6 r=4

This is the heart/lung machine which can take over the function of the heart and lungs for short periods to allow surgery to the heart itself, such as replacement of coronary artery, repair or replacement of defective heart valves, and the closing and correcting of atrial and ventricular septal defects.

The machine consists of a number of pumps, an oxygenator, a heat exchanger to control blood temperature, filters and a bubble trap. The procedure of cardiopulmonary bypass consists of inserting cannulae into the vena cava or the right atrium to take blood to the machine. The blood then flows into an oxygenator which also removes carbon dioxide and a pump then returns blood through a filter and bubble trap into a cannula connected to the aortic arch or to the femoral artery.

Clamps are placed on the aorta to isolate the heart and lungs. The heart usually arrests spontaneously. A small cannula is also required in the apex of the heart to drain blood returned from the bronchial arteries. The heat exchanger reduces the body temperature to approximately 28°C during the operation but the blood is rewarmed towards the end. Afterwards the heart may restart spontaneously or electrical defibrillation may be required.

The pumps are usually roller pumps and the oxygenator may be a bubble type or a membrane type. Further details may be found under the specific entries.

Such devices may be found in the cardiac surgery department and they are normally prepared and operated by specialized technicians (perfusionists) in conjunction with the anaesthetist.

Cardioscope n = 100 c = 3,4 r = 3

Cardioscopes are found in almost every ward and operating theatre in the hospital. They are used to show that the heart is beating, that the ECG waveform is approximately correct, and that the heart rate is reasonable. More specialized use is made of the information in coronary care units and in intensive therapy units.

In its basic form the device consists of a cathode ray tube display with associated drive circuitry, a high quality differential amplifier, a switch for selecting a small number of the standard ECG lead configurations, and a screened lead and electrodes for connection to the patient. In addition to these basic elements it may also have a small computer-type memory to retain two or three lines of the display which can be frozen and examined and also to provide a non-fading view of the last ten seconds or so of the recording. Other refinements might include a display of the average heart rate over the last few seconds, or details of the rate trend over the last few minutes or hours presented in computer-generated lettering on the same screen as the ECG. This type of computer-aided display is becoming commonplace.

Older types of cardioscope used long persistence cathode ray tubes which provided a slow moving spot with a 'comet's tail', enabling a clear view of the last few seconds of the tracing, provided the ambient light level was low.

Cardioscopes usually have a smaller bandwidth than electrocardiographs (which are used for diagnostic purposes). A typical high-frequency cut-off is 40 Hz, being sufficient to see that the main elements of the ECG waveforms are present but not sufficient for demonstrating all the possible variations from the normal. This restricted bandwidth improves noise immunity and places less demand on the quality of the electrode connections. It should be remembered here that the electrodes for cardioscopes are normally applied by the ward nursing staff, not by specialized technicians. The electrodes may be applied according to standard lead positions, but are often applied without accurate positioning, since the actual waveforms are not important.

Cardioscopes may be included in more complex diagnostic systems where heart rate and variability on a beat-to-beat basis is important. Missed beats and extra (ectopic) beats can be identified by watching the screen for every second of the day, but some cardioscopes can automatically recognize these events. Such devices might be called ectopic beat detectors, or beat-to-beat heart-rate analysers.

Cardioscopes are also used in conjunction with defibrillators, pacemakers and diathermy apparatus. In these cases the input circuitry must be capable of withstanding the relatively high voltages which may be applied directly to it. A good quality cardioscope should be able to remain connected during defibrillation or surgical diathermy without damage and with almost instant recovery of the correct display. This facility is crucial in synchronized defibrillation (see Cardioverter).

Cardiotachometer r=9

This is a device for determining heart rate. The input signal is usually the ECG; however, the arterial blood pressure wave, pulse, heart sounds or ultrasonic doppler blood flow signals may be used. There are two basic types of cardiotachometer, the averaging types which calculate the rate over a known period of time, and the beat-to-beat types which calculate the rate from the interval between each successive beat.

The averaging cardiotachometer converts the input signal to an electronic pulse corresponding to each heart beat, and these charge up a capacitor in parallel with a leak resistor. A constant rate input will cause the capacitor to charge to a steady voltage which can be applied to an indicating instrument showing heart rate. When the rate changes, the charge on the capacitor will gradually adjust to a different level. The disadvantage of this type of instrument is the insensitivity to short-term changes in rate and the long time it takes to achieve a steady state. Its advantage is its simplicity.

Beat-to-beat ratemeters work by measuring the time between each beat and then calculating the reciprocal of this time to indicate the rate. These are useful in demonstrating the erratic behaviour of the heart beat or the presence of extra or missed beats. Many cardioscopes include a cardiotachometer, presenting the rate on a meter, or as a numeric display on the cardioscope screen. Beat-to-beat ratemeters are commonly found in foetal heart monitors where changes in rate are compared with the occurrence of uterine contractions. The delays in displaying an accurate figure associated with the averaging type of ratemeter would be unacceptable in this application since the exact timing of the changes in rate must be displayed alongside the uterine contraction record.

Cardiotachometers often include alarm circuits to indicate when the rate has exceeded or gone below preset levels. Beat-to-beat ratemeters may indicate very large short-term changes in heart rate due either to extra or missed beats, or due to artefacts. Special circuits can be included to identify these three possibilities and count the number of extra beats, or suppress the rate display during artefacts.

Cardiotocograph n=10 c=4,5

This is essentially a device for recording the uterine contractions during labour. However, the term is normally applied to an instrument which also records the foetal heart rate on a beat-to-beat basis to monitor the progress of labour and in particular the wellbeing of the foetus. Uterine contractions are sometimes monitored using a tocodynamometer lightly strapped on to the mother's abdomen which consists of a central plunger coupled to a force transducer and outer guard ring so that the plunger is pressed during the uterine contractions. This provides a qualitative indication of the strength and occurrence of contractions and this is compared with the foetal heart rates which result. Sometimes an internal transducer is used once the foetal membranes have been ruptured and a recording catheter can be introduced into the uterus. The recording catheter can be a fluid-filled tube connected to an external pressure transducer or it may have a miniature pressure transducer built into the tip of the catheter.

Foetal heart rate is normally monitored by a foetal scalp electrode clamped or screwed into the foetal scalp when exposed through the opening cervix. Alternative methods of recording the foetal heart rate are to have electrodes on the mother's abdomen or an ultrasonic transducer detecting motion of the foetal heart.

The records are presented on a paper trace to identify both the effects of the contractions on foetal heart rate and the trend of these effects. In some modern instruments computer processing is applied to these signals to provide time compression to provide a display indicating the trend of these parameters during the course of labour.

Cardiotocographs are used in the labour ward but variations on these machines are used in the antenatal clinic to assess the state of the foetus in other stages of pregnancy.

Cardioverter n=15 c=4 c=3,6

Cardioversion is the correction of abnormal rhythms of the heart using a defibrillator which can be made to present its current pulse at a particular time in the cardiac cycle. They are used mainly in the coronary care unit for correcting atrial fibrillation.

The device consists of a defibrillator and an ECG monitor working through normal ECG electrodes, or detecting the ECG through the defibrillator paddles. The R wave of the ECG is identified by the monitoring circuit and used to create a triggering pulse for the defibrillator at a set (by the operator) time in the cardiac cycle.

Since cardioversion is used in circumstances where the heart is still pumping (albeit imperfectly) some skill is required to prevent the defibrillating pulse from causing fibrillation due to incorrect timing or excessive currents.

Many defibrillators intended for emergency use in cases of ventricular fibrillation also have a synchronizing facility. It is most important that the machine defaults to the asynchronous mode so that the synchronizing circuit is not used in cases of ventricular fibrillation. The use of synchronous defibrillation during ventricular fibrillation may result in failure to deliver any current, since no R wave would be detected.

Cast cutter n=5 c=1,2

Plaster casts may be removed using a pair of special shears or with an oscillating saw. This is a hand-held oscillating saw with a circular blade which, when placed on the surface of the plaster cast, will cut the hard material but will be unlikely to cause damage to the skin beneath because the oscillations are so small.

CAT scanner n=1 c=8 r=3,7

CAT stands for computerized axial tomography which relates to the assembly by computer of an image of a section through the body in line with the axis of an X-ray beam. The image displayed on the CRT screen shows relative X-ray absorption at each point in the tissue section. The device is now known as a CT scanner since it is possible to construct sections in planes other than the axial plane.

Catheter mount c=1 r=2

This is a connector which links the wide-bore corrugated breathing tube used in anaesthesia to the endotracheal connector. Both end connections are usually push fit.

Catheter puller n=1 c=3,4

A common test of urethral function in cases of urinary incontinence and urinary retention is to produce a profile of urethral closure pressure along the length of the urethra. The pressure is recorded using a tiny transducer mounted on the side or tip of the recording catheter or by using an external transducer linked to a side hole in the urethral catheter.

Devices are available to draw the catheter along the urethra at a uniform rate using a motor and gears, sometimes coupled by a cable to the point at which the catheter is gripped. In some cases an electrical signal is provided to the recording apparatus to indicate the position of the catheter to produce the profile on an $X-Y$ plotter.

Such devices are found in the urodynamic clinic which may be in the urology, gynaecology or X-ray department.

Cathode ray tube n=100 c=1,2 r=6

The most common form of display device used for the presentation of high-speed or text data is the cathode ray tube (CRT). The device, first introduced widely in the 1930s, consists of a glass envelope containing a very high vacuum in which a narrow beam of electrons is directed towards a phosphorescent screen. The electron beam is steered by electrostatic or magnetic means to cause illumination of different parts of the screen. Its real value lies in the extremely high speed by which the bright spot can be steered to different parts of the screen.

There are also specialized types of CRT (storage CRTs) used to retain the track of the bright spot. These are used in some ultrasonic scanners to build up the picture. Other types of 'non-fade' displays utilize computer memories to store the image. Most CRTs for monitoring ECG or pressure waveforms used to have long-persistence phosphors so that the path of the spot could be seen the whole way across the screen as a 'comet's tail'. These have now been largely superseded by short-persistence tubes backed up by a relatively simple computer memory to retain the whole line. Thus several cycles of a waveform are viewed clearly and this can be 'frozen' for closer examination.

Catholysis unit n=2 c=1,2

Direct electric current passing through the body causes chemical changes due to electrolysis of the salts. The effect can be used to destroy tissue selectively for the removal of hair and small skin blemishes. In these cases a large positive electrode is placed on the skin to provide a return path for the current and a negative electrode (cathode) with a small tip is applied to the point being treated. Such units may be called electrolysis or catholysis units.

Cautery unit n=10 c=3,4 r=4

This may be a separate apparatus or it may be part of an electrosurgery system. It employs a probe with a hot metal tip or wire which is used to stop bleeding and in some cases for cutting. In its very simplest form it may be a hand-held unit containing a large electrical cell which heats up a small wire loop at its tip on pressing a button. Such a unit may be used to remove very small polyps and to stop bleeding. Larger units use a low voltage source from a transformer connected to the cautery probe via a flexible lead. Very small probes exist which can be passed through an endoscope and these may include a thermocouple to allow automatic control of the tip temperature.

For cutting by wire loops a high temperature is required. For coagulation, temperatures of 100°C or so are used. Low temperatures cause deeper coagulation due to the thermal conduction in the tissue. The heat coagulation process also has the advantage of sterilizing the site of application.

Similar effects may also be caused by electrosurgery and by focused light beams and by laser light, but these are not normally called cautery.

Central venous pressure (CVP) monitor c=1 r=2,9

A long catheter is passed into a vein so that its tip lies in one of the great veins close to the heart. The pressure is usually monitored by connecting this catheter to a vertical tube fixed to a scale marked in centimetres of water pressure. The junction between the catheter and the manometer tube also connects to an intravenous fluid reservoir for flushing and body fluid replenishment. The base of the water manometer is raised to be level with the sternum.

CVP can also be monitored or recorded by connecting the catheter to a strain gauge pressure transducer and associated electronic units. CVP is measured in intensive care, open heart surgery and sometimes during anaesthesia to help assess the state of the patient or the effects of excessive positive pressure during the expiratory phase of assisted ventilation. It is also used as a guide to determine the amount of liquid a patient should receive. Normal values are in the range 3–10 cmH_2O pressure.

Centrifuge n=30 c=2,3,4

Different constituents of body fluids or body fluids mixed with reagents can be separated on the basis of their density by artificially increasing gravity in a centrifuge. The samples are mounted in tubes on a metal disc which is rotated at high speed so that the heavier components move towards the outside of the disc. Suspensions and emulsions such as blood are used so that the various component parts are separated into layers which may be identified by eye, or by a densitometer or colorimeter.

Such devices are found in the haematology department (e.g. Haematocrit centrifuge), microbiology department or sometimes on the wards. Special conditions, such as freezing, may be created in the centrifuge to favour particular reactions. The rotation speeds are sometimes very high such that special safety precautions are required to dissipate the energy of the rotor before opening the device, and special maintenance and life standards exist to avoid the possibility of failure leading to disintegration of the device.

Centrifugal analyser n=1 c=7 r=9

This is a type of automated chemical analyser used in the clinical chemistry laboratory. The basic element is a centrifuge rotor which contains a set of cuvettes around the rim which pass between the light source and photometer of a colorimeter as the disc rotates. Thus colorimetric determination of the concentration of particular chemicals in the cuvettes can be made at high speed, and sequential changes in the photometric results as the reaction in each cuvette develops may also be recorded.

The reaction in each cuvette is started as the centrifuge starts to spin. An automatic sample and diluting station loads the correct reagents and samples in separate wells on the centrifuge rotor and as the rotor starts these are drawn down and mixed in the cuvettes.

Since a complete record of the change in the photometric result from each cuvette can be logged (the starting point to the end point of the reaction in each cuvette), it is possible to identify the rate of each reaction. This is particularly useful in enzyme analysis since reaction rate is in proportion to enzyme concentration. See also Reaction rate analyser and Auto analyser.

Cerebral function monitor n=2 c=4 r=3

This is a crude form of EEG recorder using only one or two channels, which can be used in intensive care or during surgery. A slow-moving chart record is produced which displays the amplitude of the EEG over a period of time.

The higher levels of cerebral activity are taken as indicators of well-being. The absence of EEG signals may be judged to represent clinical death.

Chart recorder n=50 c=3,4 r=3

A permanent record of measurements may be required if several variables are being monitored simultaneously or the rate of change is very rapid. A chart recorder saves the information as a graph written by a pen. The chart may show the variables on the Y-axis and time on the X-axis (Y–T recorder) or two variables may be plotted against each other (X–Y recorder) on a single sheet of graph paper (as opposed to a strip of paper).

The paper strip may be driven by a motor and gearbox over a roller, sometimes with a choice of speeds. The pen(s) usually move along the vertical axis and the two main types are potentiometric and galvanometric. The pens may write using ink, or using special paper responding to pressure or heat of the pen.

Chart recorders are used to provide permanent records of ECG waveforms, blood pressures, EEG, EMG, etc. Also they are used in the pathology laboratories to record colorimetric and spectrometric information during analysis of samples.

Chart recorders may be single channel, or have up to twelve channels.

Checkerboard stimulator r=2 c=4

This provides an image in the form of a checkerboard on a screen using one or two slide projectors which alternate the black and white areas of the checkerboard, or the same effect is produced on a television image. It is used to provide the optical stimulus in the measurement of the visual evoked potential (VEP), sometimes called the visual evoked response (VER), which is a test of the detection and transmission of a light stimulus through the various stages of the eye, optic nerve, and visual cortex, as picked up from electrodes placed over the visual cortex. The VEP is measured to identify disorders of the visual system and neural disorders which may also affect the visual system.

The VEP signals are very small and it is normally necessary to employ signal averaging techniques to remove noise and artefacts. The checkerboard stimulator is triggered to change pattern at the start of the measurement cycle so that responses are synchronized in time with the stimulus, or conversely the checkerboard stimulator triggers the measurement process.

The VEP may also be measured using a flash stimulus but the reason for using a checkerboard is that there is no change in the average light level as the pattern reverses.

Chemical thermometer r=9

A clinical thermometer may be made by impregnating spots of liquid crystal material onto a spatula. If mixed with suitable dyes the transition from solid to liquid phase is demonstrated by the colour of the spot. The spots can be arranged to change colour in increments of 0.2°F over the clinical temperature range such that the number of spots changing colour indicates the temperature. Liquid crystal paints are also available which can be used to demonstrate temperature distribution by colour over parts of the body.

Chromatograph r=9

This uses a group of methods for separating a mixture of substances into their component parts. Chromatography is a misnomer for the techniques since the colour of the components is not really used for identifying substances in modern techniques. There are four basic types of chromatograph using one phase or substrate which may be liquid or solid through which the test substance (gas or liquid) moves. A common feature of these methods is that the difference in rate of movement of the components of the test sample (plus reagents) is used to identify the separate components.

In the clinical laboratory these methods are used to detect complex substances such as drugs and hormones. Examples of chromatographs are the gas–liquid chromatograph (GLC) and the thin layer chromatograph (TLC). Both these are being superseded by high-performance liquid chromatography (HPLC), although some compounds can only be measured by GLC.

Cineangiography apparatus n=1 c=7,8 r=4

This is an X-ray system producing a cine or video view of the movement of an X-ray contrast medium through the cardiovascular system. Such techniques are used to investigate arterial disease and also to provide information about the size of the chambers of the heart, the degree of pericardial, cardiac, and coronary calcification, and information about the function and haemodynamics of the heart and valves. Injection of the contrast medium into the coronary artery (cinecoronary arteriograms) may reveal the location and severity of plaque build-up. Injection just downstream to a heart valve gives an indication of the amount of regurgitation through the valve. Calculation may be made of ventricular volume and ejection fraction, assuming an ellipsoid shape at the ventricles.

Cine is normally produced on 70 mm or 105 mm film. Modern systems may include high resolution video and digital (computer aided) image enhancement.

Circle absorber n=20 c=2 r=2

During anaesthesia, the expired gases still contain some of the anaesthetic agent, and this may be rebreathed if the carbon dioxide is removed in an absorber. This is efficient in the use of anaesthetic gases, reduces pollution of the room, and raises the humidity of the inspired (rebreathed) gas.

The most commonly used rebreathing circuit is the circle closed circuit in which gases are steered round a circle of breathing tube into which is fitted a patient connection, a rebreathing bag, fresh gas inlet, and a circle absorber, including non-return valves. The absorber has a chamber full of soda-lime granules, a one-way valve and a switch to bypass the chamber. Variations on this arrangement may include two chambers for inclusion at different points in the circle, or to alternate the use of the chambers so that spent soda-lime can be bypassed in favour of a second canister. When using low flows it is essential that the circuit should be leak proof.

Clark electrode r=9

This is a polarographic electrode used for measuring the concentration of oxygen in blood and gases. The sample is brought into contact with a membrane (usually polypropylene or PTFE – Teflon) through which oxygen diffuses into a measurement chamber containing potassium chloride solution. In the chamber are two electrodes: one is a reference silver/silver chloride electrode and the other is a platinum electrode coated with glass to expose only a tiny area of platinum (e.g. 20 μm diameter). The electric current flow between the two electrodes when polarized with a voltage of 600-800 mV determines the oxygen concentration in the solution.

The reaction is very sensitive to temperature and to maintain a linear relationship between the oxygen concentration and the current measured the electrode temperature must be controlled within 0.1°C. The electrode is calibrated using two gas mixtures of known oxygen concentration. Such electrodes are used in the blood gas analyser in the clinical chemistry laboratory or in intensive care areas.

Closed circuit c=1 r=2

Although this could apply to an electrical circuit its common use in medical equipment is for an anaesthetic breathing circuit in which part or all of the expired gases are intentionally re-inspired. In such rebreathing circuits carbon dioxide is removed in an absorber. Closed circuits may be either 'to and fro' such as with the Waters canister, or 'circle' types. The advantages of the closed or partially closed circuits are that very little of the anaesthetic gases are wasted (they are rebreathed), pollution is reduced, and warming of the gases and humidification is not usually required. They are particularly attractive when using artificial ventilation.

Double pass 'to and fro' systems have the disadvantage that there is considerable dead space, there is a tendency to waterlogging, and 'channelling' may occur because the granules may shake down. They can, however, be readily sterilized. Circle systems are the most common since the dead space is reduced and the gases only make a single pass. The circle circuit conveys the gases around a circle off which there are ports for the rebreathing bag, the patient connection, and the fresh gas input. The circle absorber does not suffer from 'channelling' because of its vertical position. It can also be switched out of circuit. A vaporizer may also be included in the circuit but this must be a low resistance type, and wick types are unsuitable because of water condensation.

Cobalt-60 treatment unit n=1 c=8 r=3

Cobalt-60 produces gamma radiation at 1.17 and 1.33 MeV which is useful in the treatment of deep-seated tumours. Cobalt-60 has a half-life of 5.5 years and thus a sealed unit containing the cobalt will last for a few years. The sealed source contains a number of cobalt discs in a double stainless steel container with a brass window. The source is fitted into a treatment head which contains massive shielding (about 1 ton) and a mechanism for exposing or hiding the source by rotating it away from the collimator, or by rotating the collimator to shield the source.

The gamma-ray beam is directed at the tumour to be treated via a set of collimators and moved during the treatment so that maximum radiation dose is delivered to the point at the centre of the rotation, other parts being irradiated less.

Such devices are found in the radiotherapy department.

Cochlea implant r=4

An impression of sound, which may eventually lead to some appreciation of speech, may be achieved in totally deaf patients by the implant of an electronic stimulator connected to the auditory nerve. Experiments to date usually employ a multi-electrode bank actuated from an implant or transcutaneous wires presenting a coded signal relating to the sound reaching the external sensor.

Results with such devices show a number of difficulties and drawbacks in the translation of the technique into a clinical instrument. However, the new ability to perform high-speed coding of auditory signals through micro-computer elements offers the possibility of improvement in effectiveness.

Cold light source n=10 c=3,4

Direct viewing in the orifices and internal cavities of the body by endoscopy requires a light source. These used to be tiny bulbs mounted on the tip of the endoscope which had to work inside the body. Nearly all endoscopes now employ a flexible fibre-optic bundle to carry light from an external source to the tip of the endoscope. The instrument for providing the light is often called a cold light source. It is not in fact cold at all but is usually a high-power tungsten filament lamp with fan cooling. However, the light delivered along the endoscope is cold.

Much higher levels of illumination inside the body can be achieved using fibre-optic transmission than was previously possible, which improves the surgeon's view, and also gives a correct representation of colour. This is important in some applications (e.g. in the bladder) where diagnosis may be influenced by the colouring of the tissues examined.

Inside the light source there is a condenser and focusing system to present the light to the fibre bundle leading to the endoscope. The bundle normally has a special termination which may be a bayonet or push fit into a socket at the focal point of the lens system. Flash photography is possible if the light source contains xenon flash apparatus which can be focused onto the bundle socket.

Cold light sources are normally found in operating theatres but they may also be found in clinics where endoscopy is performed without general anaesthetic.

Collimator r=3,7

A collimator is a device for restricting and directing X-rays or other radiation by simply passing the rays through a tube (or set of parallel or divergent tubes), a cone, diaphragm, or grid made of metal which strongly absorbs the rays.

In nuclear medicine collimators are encountered as a metal, usually lead, attachment to the crystal in a gamma camera. Gamma rays are not electrically charged and so cannot be focused or directed on to the crystal, and so they are directed through a series of holes in the collimator. The rays which do not pass through holes are absorbed in the metal. A crude focusing can be effected by arranging tapered holes so that only rays from a single point can reach the crystal. The effect is enhanced by having a large number of small holes arranged in rings (e.g. 7, 19, 37, etc.) although the sensitivity may be reduced if the total surface area of hole is reduced as well. If the organ to be scanned is not at a well-defined depth a parallel hole device may be preferred, and usually a number of different collimators is available. Collimation is more effective at lower energies of rays since high-energy rays are less absorbed in the metal.

Collimators are also used in radiotherapy to confine the treatment beam to the area to be irradiated. In this case they are single-hole collimators which may also form part of an applicator to define the distance from the source to the skin.

In diagnostic radiology the X-ray set is fitted with a collimator to limit the maximum field size, and diaphragms are fitted to allow the operator to select the field size and position.

Colonoscope n=5 c=4 r=4

This is a flexible endoscope which is passed through the anus and is manipulated to view and treat sites within the colon. Viewing round corners is achieved by conveying the illumination and the image through fibre-optic bundles. The colonoscope also includes extra channels for infusing or withdrawing liquid or gas and for passing instruments for electrosurgery, cautery, and for cutting and grasping. The use of such devices has enabled viewing and treatment within the colon to be achieved without major surgery in some cases.

Colorimeter n=5 c=3,4 r=9

This is a device used in the clinical chemistry laboratory to identify the concentration of particular components of body fluids (blood, serum, urine, etc.).

There are four main components: a light source, a filter to select a particular wavelength or range of wavelengths, a sample chamber or cuvette, and a photometer. The sample of body fluid is diluted and mixed with a particular reagent to produce a coloured liquid corresponding to the colour selected by the filter. The quantity of light absorbed in the sample in the cuvette is an indication of the quantity of the chemical being tested in the sample. Colorimeters are used in automated chemical analysers to complete some of the tests, or may be separate instruments analysing single samples.

Colposcope n=5 c=4 r=4

Examination of the ovaries and fallopian tubes can be undertaken without major surgery by the use of a flexible endoscope (colposcope) passed through a very small incision in the abdominal wall. Space is created in the abdominal cavity by insufflation using carbon dioxide infused through a small channel in the colposcope. Another channel may permit the passage of small surgical instruments, notably for electrosurgery on the fallopian tubes for sterilization by causing a blockage in the tubes.

Compound (ultrasonic) scanner n=2 c=6 r=1

Ultrasonic B-scanners may provide a simple or compound scan. A simple scan provides an image which is made up of a series of parallel or diverging scan lines such that each point in the tissue is interrogated from a single direction. Most real-time scanners produce these simple scans. This has a theoretical disadvantage in that a reflecting surface which is oblique to the ultrasound beam produces an echo which is reflected away from the receiving transducer such that some reflecting surfaces may not appear on the scan image. In fact most biological surfaces are not perfect specular (mirror type) reflectors but do reflect some sound back along the line of the transmitted sound beam. Thus the images produced by simple scanners are usually satisfactory.

Compound scanners produce linear (parallel line) and sector (divergent) scans during the scanning process which are overlaid on the resulting image so that echoes are received irrespective of the orientation of the surfaces being represented. Hand-operated static B-scanners produce a compound scan which is why they are sometimes preferred to real-time scanners. See also B-scanner, Linear array scanner, Sector scanner, and Section scanner.

Computer n=20 c=3,4,5 r=3,6

Many types of computer now exist in hospitals and may include dedicated machines dealing with one job (such as calculating results from the output of a laboratory analyser) to those handling many tasks simultaneously (such as patient records and hospital financial information). The main types of computer may be classified as follows.

1. Mainframe computers. These are large digital computers usually remote from the sites of input and output and are staffed by specialist operators and programmers. They usually handle many jobs simultaneously and often in different languages and are used for financial information (salaries, sales and purchase ledgers, budgets) and for personnel and patient records.
2. Minicomputers. Usually these are in a single cabinet at the site of use and are operated by the people who require the results, although they can often be used by several people at once. Typical applications are calculating and presenting the results of dynamic isotope studies in the nuclear medicine department and for controlling process control apparatus such as the energy usage in a large hospital. Minicomputers often do the jobs which used to be performed on mainframe machines but the smaller jobs are now commonly performed on microcomputers.
3. Microcomputers. The central processor (arithmetic and logic unit) on these machines is contained on a single integrated circuit (microprocessor chip), and the whole computer (including memories, peripheral interface units and disc controllers) may be contained on a single printed circuit board. Some of these are extremely powerful and fast computers but their low cost permits them to be used on a single and often relatively trivial application such as converting the results of a single machine into a more useful form. They have an increasingly important application in the handling of text information (word processors) and at the other end of the scale may be used within medical equipment to control the operation of the equipment and manage the display of results. These are appearing

now in the most basic equipment such as infusion pumps and cardiac monitors in which they have a fixed internal program.

4. Calculators. It is not easy to draw a distinction between an electronic calculator and a microcomputer but in general a calculator is not fully programmable in that the range of functions is limited by the internal program and design, whereas a microcomputer is normally taken to mean a device which can be programmed to a variety of tasks and usually can deal with different computer languages if these are fed into it by an external device (keyboard, tape cassette, or disc drive).

5. Analogue computer. High-speed mathematical computation can be performed without converting the signals into a digital code. Instead the mathematical functions (e.g. addition, subtraction, multiplication, differentiation and integration) are performed by a series of operational amplifiers. However, the high working speeds of modern digital computers has almost removed the need for analogue machines even for real-time working such as required for process control and simulators.

Conductivity meter r=3

The concentration of an electrolyte can be measured from its electrical conductivity. This principle is used to demonstrate the purity of water, and the purity of distilled or de-ionized water is often quoted in terms of its electrical conductivity.

The technique is used extensively in haemodialysis machines to monitor the concentration of the dialysate being fed to the dialyser. Modern haemodialysis machines use a very concentrated electrolyte solution which is mixed with water at the time of use. The concentration delivered to the dialyser is critical for the correct performance of the procedure and can usually be adjusted in a proportionating pump or other mixing device. Conductivity of the mixed dialysate is usually displayed on a meter and an alarm will sound if conductivity is too high or too low. Typical concentration limits are from 130 to 145 mmol/l of sodium.

These devices are incorporated into the haemodialysis machine but the service technician would normally also have a calibrated test instrument through which the dialysate can be passed to verify the performance of the internal monitoring system.

Constant voltage transformer n=5 c=3

Some electrical apparatus is very sensitive to changes in the mains supply voltage. This is particularly important where the mains supply is erratic to the extent that the performance or quality of the results from the apparatus may be impaired. A constant voltage transformer has compensating windings to allow a relatively steady output voltage during fluctuations of the input voltage within a limited range. Most apparatus is developed and produced in countries which have reliable electrical supplies and so the design is often unsatisfactory for more erratic supplies.

Continuous ambulatory peritoneal dialysis (CAPD) r=3

Peritoneal dialysis can sometimes be used as an alternative to haemodialysis and uses the natural membrane of the peritoneum. This is a double membrane which envelops most of the organs in the abdomen. A soft tube (usually silicon rubber) is surgically inserted through the skin into the space between the two membranes and through which a special sterile dialysing fluid is passed. Toxins of small molecular weight will pass into the dialysing fluid and it is then withdrawn and new fluid passed in again.

Although this technique has been used for many years with a system of valves and timers and a heater to control the change of fluid, a new technique is gaining popularity which allows the patient much more freedom. In continuous ambulatory peritoneal dialysis a collapsible bag which contains about two litres of the fluid is connected to the tube leading to the peritoneum. The fluid is discharged from the bag through the tube and the bag is then folded up onto a belt worn by the patient. After a few hours the fluid is returned to the bag, and a new bag fitted when required.

The value of this technique is that it gives the patient much greater freedom, and is less susceptible to infection due to less frequent connection and disconnection. The quality of the dialysate is much more important than in haemodialysis since it does come into direct contact with the patient tissues.

Continuous flow analyser n=2 c=5,6,7 r=9

This is one type of automated chemical analyser which may be used in the clinical chemistry laboratory to estimate the concentration of a range of ions and molecules found in samples of body fluids such as blood and urine.

The basic technique is to move the sample to be tested (usually in diluted form), together with a quantity of a reagent, along a narrow tube to a colorimeter which will identify the original concentration from the optical density of the sample. The chemical reaction necessary to produce the result takes place as the bolus of fluid passes along the tube. Special conditions may be created if the particular analytical process requires it, such as heating, or introducing the sample to the reagent via a dialyser if other constituents of the sample might interfere with the reaction.

Each bolus of fluid is separated from the next by a bubble of air which acts to clean the inside of the tube and prevent contamination of one sample by the next. Usually samples alternate with a washing mixture so that this separation is optimized.

Several tests may be carried out at the same time using separate tubes and processes according to the test being performed. An example of a continuous flow analyser is the Technicon SMA (sequential multiple analyser) series which may perform six or twelve separate tests at the same time. Later versions are able to analyse 20 parameters on 0.4 ml samples at a rate of 150 samples/hour.

This type of analyser is very popular. Its main disadvantage is that every available test is normally performed on every sample, with resultant (sometimes unnecessary) cost.

The addition of a computer enables an extension of the automatic process to the printing and mailing of the results or direct communication over computer lines.

Coolidge tube r=3

This is a stationary anode X-ray tube which was the fore runner of the modern X-ray tube. It consists of an envelope, usually glass, in which there is a heated tungsten filament and focusing electrode from which electrons are attracted to a copper anode maintained at a high (kV) voltage, and into which is embedded a tungsten target. X-rays are produced when the electrons are stopped by the target. The efficiency of X-ray production is only about 1% and so there is the major problem of disposing of the remaining (heat) energy. Various designs of cooling mechanism are in use, some of which use oil cooling, since this also provides a good insulator for the very high voltages (up to 500 kV) which are required. To limit the voltage employed the cathode and anode are often maintained at equal negative and positive voltages.

Stationary anode tubes are now only found in small X-ray units (e.g. portable and dental).

Copper kettle (vaporizer) n=2 c=1 r=2

A way of dealing with the variation in the concentration of anaesthetic vapours due to temperature change (caused by rapid loss of latent heat of vaporization), and caused by variations in the gas flow, were dealt with in a simple way in 'copper kettle' type vaporizers such as the Halox. The temperature problem is dealt with by thermal damping either by copper, hot water (e.g. Oxford vaporizer), or by electricity (e.g. Heidbrink Kinet-O-Meter). Variations in gas flow are not a problem since a small quantity of oxygen from a separate rotameter is saturated with vapour (i.e. concentration is known) and this carrier mixture is fed into the main anaesthetic gas

67

flow. Unlike most vaporizers now in use, the result is a known delivery rate of the agent and not a known percentage of a variable gas flow.

Most copper kettle vaporizers employ a gauze or mesh in the liquid through which the gas is bubbled.

Coulter counter n=3 c=5,6 r=9

This is a trade name for a particle counter which calculates a number of characteristics of blood samples, and is used in the haematology department. The essential element in the device is a cell counter (haemocytometer) which causes blood cells to pass through a small aperture through which an electric current is being passed between electrodes each side of the aperture. As a cell passes through there will be a transient change in the electrical resistance since the resistance of a blood cell will be higher than the electrolyte in which it is suspended.

There are various types of Coulter counter classified according to the number of analyses performed. A useful example is the model 'S' in which the sample of blood is diluted in a ratio of 1:224 and then split into two separate channels, one for determining the white cell count and haemoglobin content, and the other for determining the red cell count. In the first channel a lysing agent is added to break down the red blood cells (from which the haemoglobin content is calculated by spectrophotometric methods) and the white cells are counted in an aperture device as described above, usually with three separate channels which should all agree within a defined margin for the final result. The second channel undergoes further dilution because of the high red blood cell count and is then fed to a similar three aperture device for counting the cells. The model 'S' contains a calculating module which uses these results to determine a number of commonly used indices of blood composition including the mean corpuscular volume (MCV), haematocrit, mean corpuscular haemoglobin (MCH), mean corpuscular haemoglobin concentration (MCHC), etc.

There are other types of haemocytometer which utilize optical detection of the passage of cells through the gate such as the Fisher autocytometer.

Cryosurgery apparatus n=6 c=4 r=4

A metallic probe making contact with the tissue is cooled to a very low temperature (e.g. $-196°C$ for liquid nitrogen). The effect is to freeze the surrounding tissue so that it dies. In the tissue immediately beyond the killed zone a degree of coagulation occurs thus limiting the resulting bleeding. The technique is used for freezing and breaking off small polyps, and also for resecting the prostate gland. For larger lesions liquid nitrogen cooling is required since a large ice ball is necessary. Other cryogenic surgery devices utilize the Joule–Thomson effect, usually by the expansion of nitrous oxide from a cylinder through an orifice in the tip of the probe, although low power types for ophthalmology use carbon dioxide.

In devices using liquid nitrogen a dewar or thermos bottle is required as a reservoir from which the liquid is piped to the probe and the resulting boiled-off gas drawn off through a tube. In order to localize the cooling at the tip, the shank of the probe may contain a heater to prevent freezing of tissue distal to the treatment site. Gas expansion devices are relatively easy to control by interrupting the gas flow but they cannot remove heat at the rate achieved with liquid nitrogen.

They are used in operating theatres, special clinics and chiropody clinics.

Cryotherapy apparatus r=4

Cold therapy may be applied using vapour coolants, ice, ice-water or cold packs for the treatment of acute soft tissue trauma, such as sprains and strains of muscle or tendon. In the case of sprays, ethyl chloride may be sprayed on to the skin and cooling is effected by evaporation. This is highly inflammable, and so precautions must be taken to eliminate fire hazards. Conductive cooling is the most widely used method, using ice or an antifreeze mixture applied to the skin for treatment periods of thirty minutes or so. Such methods would be used in the physiotherapy department.

CT scanner n=1 c=8 r=3,7

Previously called the EMI scanner, and the CAT scanner, this is now known as the CT (computerized tomography) scanner. It produces an image on a CRT screen of a section through the body, with each point on the image having a brightness corresponding to the X-ray absorption properties of the point represented.

The scanner comprises one or more X-ray sources collimated to produce very thin X-ray beams which pass through the patient to a scintillation detector. The overall attenuation of the X-ray beam as it passes through the body is calculated from the intensity reaching the detector. Similar attenuation measurements are made thousands of times as the position and direction of the X-ray beam is changed. A computer with suitable programs calculates the attenuation occurring at each point within the section being scanned which would be necessary to account for the measured overall attenuations. A variety of different scanning methods, and arrangements of single or multiple heads and/or detectors, are in use.

The first and probably most important use of CT scanners was in brain scanning, but they are also used widely for imaging all parts of the body. An important advantage over conventional X-ray techniques is that soft tissues can be clearly seen and differentiated. A major improvement in recent years has been in the number of elements which can be resolved in the image, and shorter scanning times. Other developments have allowed the presentation of tomographic planes other than the axial section.

Cuirass ventilator n=0 c=3 r=2

As its name implies, this machine takes the form of a breast plate. A rigid dome fits over the chest and air is pumped to make the chest wall rise and fall. This provides only a limited assistance to the lungs but has proved useful for patients in transit, in poliomyelitis and in domiciliary treatment. There is a variation on this device using a rubber bag, called the Pinkerton cuirass ventilator.

Culdoscope

This is a special gynaecological type of endoscope for viewing into the pouch of Douglas, the ovaries and fallopian tubes. It is a rigid tube which is passed into the vagina and makes a puncture through the posterior wall into the space beyond. These are not often used now since the laparoscope, which is passed through the abdominal wall, has been found more satisfactory.

Current bath n=1 c=2 r=10

Electrical stimulation of the muscles as a form of physiotherapy is normally applied through electrodes mounted on the skin over the muscles concerned. A more general stimulation, often intended to improve blood supply, may be achieved by immersing a limb in a special water bath in which the electrodes are placed but without contacting the limb. Faradic and sinusoidal stimulating currents may be used and the application may be bipolar or monopolar. In a bipolar bath treatment electrodes are placed each side of, or at each end of, the limb to be treated whereas in monopolar baths one electrode may be placed directly on the limb. Treatment is normally performed in water without the addition of salt so that more of the current will pass through the limb itself.

The apparatus used with current baths is the same as for electrotherapy using surface electrodes, i.e. faradic treatment unit or electrotherapy set.

Cuvette r=9

In clinical chemistry tests are performed using a spectrometer or other device to detect the absorption or emission of light of particular wavelengths from a sample of a body fluid, on its own or in conjunction with a reagent.

The cuvette is the glass or plastic optical chamber in which the absorption or emission is tested. The design and expense involved in the cuvette design may determine the overall accuracy.

Cystometer n=3 c=4

A cystometer measures the pressure in the bladder as it fills. Although this could theoretically be performed during natural filling, it is normally performed by infusing water or saline through a urethral catheter. Cystometry is an important diagnostic test in the investigation of urinary incontinence or retention.

Cystometers can be purchased as independent instruments comprising a strip chart recorder, a pressure measuring device connected to the chart recorder, and an infusion pump or infusion controller to deliver the fluid. The result is a graph of pressure against volume known as a cystometrogram. The normal result shows little or no rise in pressure during filling (0–15 cmH_2O pressure up to 500 ml in adults) whereas some abnormal results show involuntary contractions of the bladder.

Modern cystometers are electronic and usually infuse water or saline but other types do exist which are mechanical, using aneroid pressure measuring devices and/or infusing carbon dioxide rather than a liquid. Cystometry is more commonly performed using a polygraph on which other tests and recordings are made. Additional recordings may include rectal pressure, urethral pressure and flow, flow velocity during voiding, and electromyography of the urethral sphincter or adjacent muscles.

Such apparatus would be used by urologists or gynaecologists in the X-ray suite or in a special 'urodynamics' clinic.

Cystoscope n=20 c=3,4 r=4

This is a telescope less than a centimetre in diameter which may be passed through the urethra for viewing inside the bladder. Extra open channels through the telescope may be used for sampling fluid in the bladder or ureters, or special manipulating instruments may be used for electrosurgery or for grasping, cutting or crushing material within the bladder or on the bladder wall. Cystoscopes are usually rigid tubes with light supplied via a fibre-optic bundle and may also convey the image to the eyepiece via a coherent fibre-optic bundle. Older types use a small electric bulb at the tip.

D

De-aerator r=3

This is a device or mechanism for removing air from liquids, and is found in haemodialysis machines.

Dialysing fluid passes through an artificial kidney at a lower pressure than the blood on the other side of the membrane, especially if water is to be removed from the patient by ultrafiltration. The low pressure of the dialysing fluid causes release of dissolved air which may pass through the dialyser into the blood. The de-aerator removes the air before the fluid reaches the dialyser, and it does this by lowering the pressure and/or raising the temperature in the chamber before the dialyser.

Defibrillator n=20 c=4 r=3,6

Heart disease, electrolyte disturbances, or electric shock, can cause the normally co-ordinated action of the ventricular heart muscle to be disrupted. The unco-ordinated contractions of different parts of the ventricles is called ventricular fibrillation which may lead to death within a few minutes. The most effective treatment for this condition is to pass a short pulse of electrical current through the ventricles. This is done after open heart surgery by applying electrodes directly to the heart. In all other situations (external defibrillation) electrodes are applied to the chest and a large current (e.g. 50 A for 5 ms) is required for this.

A defibrillator employs a high-voltage generator to charge a capacitor to a high voltage, up to 7 kV. This capacitor is discharged into the body via two large electrodes placed across the axis of the heart or between the back and front of the chest. The electrodes (called paddles) are coated with conductive electrode jelly and are spring loaded and shaped to prevent the jelly spreading to the handgrips. There is also an inductor placed between the capacitor and the electrodes to produce a damped sinusoidal waveform which has been found to give good results. Some machines produce other waveforms (e.g. trapezoidal).

The typical maximum stored energy in the capacitor is 400 J, but low energy is normally used for the first attempt and then increased at each subsequent attempt until success is achieved. This is because excessive energy may cause damage to the heart, and burn the skin at the electrode sites. For children, and for use with internal electrodes (i.e. directly applied to the heart) the stored energy required may be only 50 J. Most defibrillators have a safety interlock so that energy is limited to this level when used with internal electrodes.

Older types of defibrillator (now obsolete) used a short burst of alternating current applied directly from a large mains transformer. These are now considered to be dangerous.

The ECG may be recorded through the defibrillator paddles and it is now common for defibrillators to have an integral ECG monitor, allowing proper diagnosis of ventricular fibrillation to be made and an immediate confirmation of success or failure of the procedure. An ECG recorder may also be provided. The ECG monitor is particularly important when defibrillators are used to correct abnormal rhythms of the heart rather than ventricular fibrillation. In this case the defibrillating pulse must be applied at the correct time in the cardiac cycle and hence these types are called synchronized defibrillators or cardioverters which take the R wave of the ECG signal, apply a delay which can be set by the operator and then deliver the current pulse. Incorrect timing of the pulse can damage the heart or cause ventricular fibrillation.

Defibrillator tester n=5 c=1,2 r=3,6

Defibrillators need checking frequently since they may only be used occasionally (e.g. once a year) but must function perfectly when required. Testers are available which consist of a large (usually 50 Ω) non-inductive resistor connected to metal plates on to which the defibrillator paddles may be pressed. The action of the defibrillator is confirmed by the flash of a neon lamp connected across a low value resistor in series with the load resistor or there may be a meter to display the energy delivered in joules. A more complicated tester is required to confirm the correct action of a synchronized defibrillator (cardioverter).

De-ionizer n=20 c=2 r=3

Impurities in water may be removed by a water softener or by a de-ionizer. These are most commonly encountered in connection with haemodialysis in which the concentration and composition of the dialysing fluid is extremely important, particularly if the life of the patient is sustained by haemodialysis for long periods. A de-ionizer is required in place of a water softener if there are significant quantities of calcium or magnesium in the domestic water supply. Aluminium levels exceeding 0.06 ppm can also cause serious disorders following long-term dialysis.

The de-ionizer employs an ion exchange resin column through which the water passes and this must be returned to the manufacturer or replaced at frequent intervals, which is relatively expensive. Automatic changeover systems also exist.

Delayed auditory feedback machine n=2 c=2,3

The rhythm of speech can be affected by amplifying the sound of one's own voice, and delaying its presentation. Delayed auditory feedback machines exist which present the subject's own voice via headphones, and controls on the unit allow variation in the amplitude and time delay. The technique is used in the speech therapy department for the treatment of stammering and speech-rhythm disorders.

Demand flow analgesia apparatus n=50 c=3 r=2

For analgesia during labour, emergency surgery and dental surgery it is common to use a demand flow, or intermittent flow machine. A bag or reservoir is filled with the required gases (usually nitrous oxide and oxygen) at slightly above atmospheric pressure, and the patient inhales this gas via a low-pressure valve on demand. Some machines such as the Entonox apparatus use a premixed gas from a cylinder, while others such as the Walton 5, Mckesson, Lucy Baldwyn, AE, and Quantiflex RA actually mix the gases to a formula determined by control settings.

Demand flow systems may also include a low-resistance vaporizer in a draw-over circuit.

Densitometer n=5 c=2,4 r=3,7,9

This measures the optical density of items placed between a light source and a light detector. Optical density is expressed as follows:

$$D = \log_{10} I_1/I_r$$

where D is the optical density, I_1 is the light detected through the test material and I_r is the light detected directly.

Densitometers are common in the pathology laboratory for reading acetate electrophoretic strips. In this case the strip is moved through the light beam and a profile of the optical density along the strip is produced on a chart. The peaks of density recorded in this way represent particular materials in the original test samples.

Densitometers are also used on photographic and X-ray film. For instance, an X-ray film badge contains a small photographic film, and after development the optical density of each part of it is measured to determine radiation exposure. A densitometer may also be found in the X-ray department or used by the X-ray service engineer for checking X-ray set and film processor performance. Typical values for the density of exposed X-ray film might be 0.1 (fog level) up to 3.0 (darkest area).

Depilator n=1 c=2

For removal of hairs, usually by electrolysis (catholysis), a fine metal probe is brought into contact with the base of a hair and a direct electrical current is passed through. Chemical changes caused by the current in the vicinity of the probe tip cause the hair follicle to die. The probe forms the negative electrode (cathode) and the positive electrode is attached to the skin nearby. The positive electrode has a large surface area so that the current density beneath it never reaches toxic levels. The same instrument may sometimes be called an electrolysis unit, catholysis unit, or epilation unit.

Dialysate conductivity meter n=5 c=3 r=3,9

Every haemodialysis machine contains this device which monitors the concentration of the fluid being delivered to the dialyser by measuring its electrical conductivity. The equipment service technician may also carry a conductivity meter as a test instrument.

Dialysate pressure monitor r=3

This device monitors the negative pressure of the dialysate fluid on one side of the dialyser membrane. Control of fluid removal from the patient's blood is effected by adjusting the suction created by an effluent pump. The pressure settings are monitored, usually within the main console of the haemodialysis machine, to prevent insufficient or excessive fluid removal.

Dialysate proportionating pump

Most haemodialysis machines use a reservoir of a concentrated dialysate with purified tap water added to create the concentration required for passing through the artificial kidney. This is achieved in a proportionating pump which draws in the concentrate and tap water, and produces the correct mixture. The pump has a motor and gear train driving a double pump chamber, one for the dialysate concentrate, and the other for water, and the relative volumes of these chambers can be adjusted to change the mixing ratio.

Dialyser n=20 c=1,4 r=3

The main element in a dialyser is a semipermeable membrane through which small molecules can pass by diffusion. Dialysers are encountered in medical work in renal dialysis where unwanted small molecules (e.g. urea) and water can be removed from the body. Dialysers may also be encountered in the clinical chemistry laboratory for purifying or modifying samples of fluid being analysed.

Haemodialysers (sometimes called artificial kidneys) take blood from the body and pass it along one side of the dialysing membrane so that unwanted small molecules may diffuse into a special dialysing fluid passing along the other side. Small molecules which need not be removed are included in the dialysate so that there is equal diffusion of these molecules in each direction.

Haemodialysers are constructed either as membranes wound into coils (not used now), membranes held between flat plates, or made into hollow fibres along the length of a special vessel.

The peritoneum is a double membrane enveloping most of the organs in the abdomen, and renal dialysis may be achieved by pumping a special dialysing fluid into the cavity between the two membranes and allowing time for the diffusion to occur before withdrawing it. This technique is called peritoneal dialysis which may be a hospital procedure operated by sets of pumps, valves and timers, or may be used at the patient's home without special apparatus but using a collapsible bag from which the fluid is delivered and then returned after the process is complete. Both dialysis systems have their advantages.

Dialyser washout device n=20 c=2

Early types of haemodialyser (e.g. Kiil) required reconstruction with new membranes each time they were used (two to three times per patient per week). Now, disposable dialysers are available which are more satisfactory in a number of ways, but the costs are high. Devices can be purchased which 'wash out' used disposable dialysers so that they can be reused a number of times. These usually consist of a set of valves and timers which provide a programme of washing and disinfection for the used dialyser.

Dialysis clamp

Peritoneal dialysis as performed in hospitals often requires an electrical or electronic device to control the flow of fluid into the potential space between the membranes of the peritoneum and to draw off the spent fluid after a period of time. The dialysis clamp therefore clamps off the outlet tube while the fluid is being infused, and clamps the inlet tube whilst fluid is being discharged to waste. The device itself consists of electronic or electrical timers and electromechanical gate valves.

Diathermy equipment n=20 c=4 r=3,4

Diathermy means internal heating where the heat is generated by a direct conversion to heat of some other form of energy passing through the tissues. In the case of surgical diathermy as used in the operating theatre for cutting and coagulating tissue an electric current passes through the body and heat is generated by resistive loss. In short-wave or microwave diathermy as used in the physiotherapy department, heating is caused by the dielectric loss of the tissues when electromagnetic waves pass through (the same effect as used in microwave ovens). Diathermy can also be produced by the absorption of ultrasonic waves, and this effect is also employed in the physiotherapy department.

In the case of surgical diathermy, high-frequency electric current is made to pass through the body between two contact electrodes. High frequencies (0.5 to 3.0 MHz) are used because direct current, or low-frequency alternating current (e.g. the 50 Hz or 60 Hz of the mains supply) would cause muscle spasm. Bipolar diathermy (less often used) causes the current to pass between the two arms of a special forceps so that tissue held between the tips is heated causing the death of the tissue and the cessation of bleeding. In the more conventional monopolar diathermy one electrode is large (e.g. 100 cm^2) and attached to the skin whilst the other is a pointed or ball-tipped probe held in contact with the tissue to be cut or coagulated. This causes intense heating at the point of contact between the probe and the tissue since the current density is very high. Little or no heating is produced at the large electrode because the current density is low. The large and small electrodes are known as the indifferent (or dispersive), and active electrodes respectively. The current generators for surgical diathermy may be spark gap types (very old), valve (old) or transistor. Since the current generated is in the radio-frequency part of the electromagnetic spectrum they can cause widespread interference with other electronic equipment in or near the operating theatre (e.g. EEG equipment).

Diathermy equipment used in the physiotherapy department usually involves the production of an electrostatic field in the body from two large (e.g. 10 cm diameter) electrodes placed each side of the body and operating at 27 MHz. Other types direct microwave radiation at the skin to produce a more superficial heating. Both types cause mild internal heating from which the therapeutic effect is derived.

Ultrasound is absorbed by living tissues to a varying degree depending on the frequency employed (the higher the frequency the greater the proportion of energy absorbed), and the type of tissue. They are used with frequencies in the range 1–3 MHz and total power of 1–3 W to cause heating of tissue (particularly joint capsules) where the heating is said to speed repair processes and relieve inflammation. See also entries on Surgical diathermy, Short-wave and Microwave diathermy, and Ultrasonic diathermy.

Diathermy tester n=1 c=2,3

The output power of surgical diathermy apparatus may need testing as part of the servicing procedure. In its simplest form the tester may consist of a group of lightbulbs, possibly with a light cell to measure the light output. A more precise measurement may be made using a large non-inductive resistor and a radio-frequency ammeter calibrated in output power. A typical output for a surgical diathermy apparatus is 200 W but more powerful devices suitable for underwater surgery in the bladder may deliver up to 800 W. Diathermy testers would be found in the electronics laboratory. Testers also exist for short-wave diathermy apparatus, of the type used in the physiotherapy department.

Differential amplifier r=3

Most amplifiers deal with signals which exist between a signal wire and ground. Differential amplifiers, which are widely used in ECG, EEG, EMG, and pressure amplifiers are intended to amplify the difference in voltage between two signal lines and should ignore any voltage which exists simultaneously on the two signal lines (the common mode signal). The most common common-mode signal is 50 Hz (or 60 Hz) pick-up which may be several volts in some situations, whereas the differential signal may be measured in microvolts in the case of the EEG. Thus a good differential amplifier must have a high common mode rejection ratio (CMRR) of the order of 80 to 100 dB.

CMRR is degraded if the source impedance is different on each signal lead (such as in the case of skin electrodes with unequal quality of application) and so CMRR is usually quoted for a particular source impedance inequality (e.g. 5000 Ω).

Discrete sample analyser n=1 c=7,8 r=9

This is a type of automated chemical analyser used in the clinical chemical laboratory for the estimation of concentrations of various ions, molecules and enzymes in samples of body fluids. The discrete analyser may be distinguished from continuous flow analysers and from centrifugal analysers in that the particular tests and chemical procedures required are programmed for each sample. In general the diluted sample undergoes all the reactions required in the same cuvette which is eventually fed to the photometer for the final analysis. Discrete sample analysers would be difficult to operate without computers. Their main advantage is economy of reagents since only the tests which have been requested need be performed.

Dispersive electrode r=4

This is another term used for the indifferent electrode applied to the buttocks or strapped round the leg during electrosurgery (surgical diathermy) to draw off the current applied to the surgical site by an active electrode.

Doppler blood flow/velocity meter n=2 c=3,4 r=1,3

Flow velocity in blood vessels can be estimated from outside the body using ultrasound. An ultrasonic transducer comprising two small piezoelectric elements, one for transmit and one for receive, is placed on the skin over the blood vessel in question so that a narrow beam of continuous wave ultrasound passes through it. Some of the energy is back-scattered to the receiving transducer from the blood and the frequency of the returning waves is shifted in frequency (by the doppler effect) in proportion to the velocity of the blood. Unfortunately blood flow is complicated by the fact that it is pulsatile, and because the velocity is not uniform across the vessel (velocity is higher at the centre). Thus there are many different frequencies in the returning signals and these are changing rapidly.

To calculate the blood flow velocity the mean frequency of the doppler signal can be calculated and this is related to mean blood velocity. The mean frequency can be obtained using analogue circuits or a spectrum analyser and computer. Absolute measurement of velocity is difficult because the angle between the blood flow and ultrasound beam is not known, and flow rate calculation requires a knowledge of the internal diameter of the vessel. The zero-crossing detector provides a simple and inexpensive method of obtaining a rough estimate of flow velocity.

The main use of such systems is in detecting flow abnormalities in peripheral arteries occurring in disease of the vascular system. Although the methods are imperfect, they are sometimes more desirable than using X-ray contrast techniques (which show the anatomy) because of the risks and pain associated with invasive procedures.

Doppler blood flow signals can now be linked to ultrasonic B-scanning so that the image formed is gated to show only those parts of the anatomy which are moving. The image formed has some of the advantages of X-ray imaging but is safer to obtain and can provide quantitative information about the flow patterns at particular points on the image. Arterial strictures can be identified thus reducing the need for exploratory surgery and also permitting the repeated assessment of the diseased artery after treatment.

DOPPLER FOETAL HEART DETECTOR/MONITOR

A typical system might include the transducer, a high-frequency oscillator (typically between 5 and 15 MHz), a receiving amplifier, a detector (often bi-directional), a frequency spectrum analyser, and a meter, display or recording device. They would be found in the surgical ward or a special vascular diagnostic clinic.

Doppler foetal heart detector/monitor n=10 c=2,4 r=1

Movement of the foetal heart and blood in the foetal and placental circulation can be detected with an ultrasonic doppler device which has a transducer placed on the skin containing two ultrasonic crystals. One transmits a continuous wave ultrasonic beam into the body and the other detects returning echoes. The echoes from moving structures are shifted in frequency and this shift is detected and delivered to a loudspeaker or applied to a pattern recognition circuit which identifies the beats of the heart.

In its simplest form (the foetal heart detector) the doppler frequencies are applied to a loudspeaker and give an indication of foetal life and the foetal heart rate. These are used extensively in the antenatal clinic and sometimes in the labour ward. These devices comprise the transducer, an oscillator operating at the ultrasonic frequency (usually around 2 MHz), a tuned amplifier, and a simple demodulation circuit followed by an audio amplifier and loudspeaker.

The foetal heart monitor is used during labour to record the foetal heart rate on a chart alongside a second trace showing the uterine contractions. Well-known patterns of foetal heart rate variation occur in response to the uterine contractions and abnormalities in these patterns indicate foetal distress. The transducer used for the foetal heart rate monitor is different from those used on the simple detectors in that the transmitted beam has a wide angle to guarantee that ultrasonic waves pass through the foetal heart even when the foetus has moved, and there are a number of receiving crystals facing in different directions to ensure detection of returning echoes from the foetus at all times. Not all foetal heart rate monitors employ ultrasound since the preferred method is to detect the foetal heart rate from the foetal ECG.

Doppler (ultrasonic) blood pressure monitor n=3 c=4 r=1

Arterial blood pressure has a peak (systolic) pressure occurring when the heart pumps and a trough (diastolic) just before the next pumping stroke. These two pressures are commonly identified in the operating theatre, ward, clinic or doctor's surgery using a sphygmomanometer. In this case an inflatable cuff is placed around the upper arm and the pressure in the cuff inflated above the systolic pressure (typically 120 mmHg) and then slowly released as sounds from the artery downstream of the cuff are detected using a stethoscope placed on the lower arm. The systolic pressure is identified as blood first begins to spurt through the artery which has been held closed by the cuff pressure. The diastolic pressure is identified by a different sound when the artery is just failing to close.

The stethoscope can be replaced by a thin ultrasonic transducer placed under the inflatable cuff which detects the movement of the artery wall. The doppler signals are detected and fed to a pattern recognition circuit which identifies the characteristic signals occurring as the cuff pressure falls past the systolic and diastolic pressures.

These devices are claimed to be more accurate than alternative (acoustic) methods when the pulse is weak, or when there is patient movement or high background noise.

The device contains a double piezoelectric transducer (one section for receive, the other for transmit) coupled to the skin with a jelly, an oscillator to energize the transmit transducer, a receiving amplifier, and a doppler detector and pattern recognition circuit. Sometimes the pressures are recorded on a paper chart to monitor the trend.

Doppler ultrasonic scanner n=1 c=6 r=1

Information about the motion of blood in the larger vessels may be obtained from the doppler shifted reflections received by a transducer outside the body. This is most commonly used to assess the quality of flow from an audible signal produced from the doppler shifted components or by processing of these signals to indicate the flow pattern or flow rate. Images can also be produced by combining the information derived from these doppler signals with B-scan images. There are two main types.

A continuous wave doppler transducer may be scanned back and forth across the skin and an image produced corresponding to the scan plane, which writes on the screen only when doppler signals are being received. Thus a plan of blood vessels immediately beneath the transducer may be produced.

A more complex type exists in which the continuous wave is interrupted to form short bursts of ultrasound which interrogate small sections of the tissue beneath the transducer in sequence. By moving the transducer across the skin a B-scan is produced. However, the B-scan is gated to prevent the presentation of any echoes arising from tissue which is not moving. In this way a section scan is produced showing only those sites which exhibit motion. The doppler signals also contain information about the flow rate at each moving point on the image and this may be presented on a colour display which shows different flow rates as different colours. This is particularly useful since a diseased artery will have turbulent flow (or flow separation) in which flow may exist in both directions at once. The colour display can provide unequivocal evidence of arterial disease and identify the site of any constriction or dilatation.

Such techniques are used by vascular surgeons in special clinics and they offer the potential of avoiding dangerous and painful X-ray contrast procedures.

Dose-rate meter n=2 c=3,4 r=7

This is a device intended to show the radiation dose-rate occurring in an X-ray beam. Since dose rate (rads/min) is the rate of X-ray absorption, a dose-rate meter is in fact no more than an exposure meter. The dose-rate is inferred from the exposure.

Exposure rate is sensed in an ionization chamber or scintillator, and such devices are used in radiation protection monitoring or in the X-ray department for personnel monitoring and equipment performance checking.

Dosemeter/dosimeter n=2 c=2,3,4 r=7

This is a device for calculating the X-ray exposure, at a point within an X-ray beam. The desired quantity is often X-ray dose (rads) but since dose calculation requires information about X-ray absorption in the tissues, dose can only be inferred.

Dosimeters detect the radiation using ionizing chambers, photographic methods, scintillators, or indirectly using thermoluminescent devices. Dosimetry systems and equipment exist within hospitals in radiation protection, nuclear medicine, radiotherapy, and X-ray departments for use in personnel monitoring and X-ray set peformance checking.

Drager volumeter n=10 c=2 r=6

This is similar to the Wright's respirometer and is a small dial gauge which fits into an anaesthetic or ventilator circuit for measuring gas flow. See Wright's respirometer.

Draw-over apparatus r=2

The main object of a draw-over apparatus is to enable a volatile anaesthetic agent to be vaporized in air with complete independence from supplies of nitrous oxide and oxygen. Air is drawn through a vaporizer by the patient's breathing effort. These devices may include simple ether vaporizers such as the Schimmelbusch mask, or low-resistance vaporizers such as the AE, Blease universal, EMO ether vaporizer, etc. They are often used in

82

conjunction with demand flow anaesthesia or analgesia apparatus such as the Walton 5, McKesson, Lucy Baldwyn and Quantiflex RA system.

Draw-over vaporizer n=5 c=2 r=2

An anaesthetic vaporizer with a low resistance to the flow of gas is required in some circumstances, particularly where gas is drawn through the vaporizer by the effort of the patient, or where it is included in the anaesthetic circuit. These are relatively common in dental anaesthesia and in portable emergency apparatus. Examples of these are the Blease Universal vaporizer, which can be used with a variety of agents, and the Oxford Miniature vaporizer, the Rowbottom, AE, the Goldman, Enfluratec 5%, Fluotec 5%, Tritec 1.5% and Ethertec 5%.

Drinker apparatus r=4

This is the original 'iron lung' device to generate a negative pressure around the thorax of the patient to cause inflation of the lungs when the normal breathing process is defective such as in polio.

Drop counter/ratemeter n=20 c=2

Gravity-fed fluid infusion systems are normally set up by the nurse by checking the drop rate in the giving set drip chamber against a watch. Many infusion pumps and controllers use the drop rate (detected optically) to determine the quantity of fluid being infused, and devices now exist simply to detect and display the drop rate without actually controlling the flow.

The devices are relatively small in size and clip on to the drip chamber, and contain an electronic circuit to calculate the drop rate and present it on a digital display. The devices are useful in the setting up of drip systems, and also in longer-term monitoring of the drip rate.

Drop detector head

It is now common to control the delivery of intravenous fluids automatically using a pump or automatic controller. The most common method of detecting the quantity of fluid being infused is an optical gate clamped on to the drip chamber on the standard fluid infusion set. The gate consists of a collimated light source on one side of the drip chamber and a photoelectric detector on the other. As the drop falls through the light beam a pulse is presented to the controller and is counted. In the case of the automatic controllers (as opposed to pumps) a valve opens to allow a number of drops fall through. If this exceeds the number allowed in the time which has elapsed, the gate valve closes for a time. The flow is not steady, but the total quantity of fluid infused over several minutes will be correct.

Problems are often experienced with this type of detector head because of the effects of extraneous light (e.g. sunlight) and incorrect positioning on the drip chamber. Some equipment manufacturers insist on a specific type of infusion set being used to minimize this problem. Another problem is that the number of drops in 1 ml of fluid differs for each type of drip set and infusion fluid. Also the fluid used and the temperature, etc. can affect the amount delivered. If the infusion rate rises accidentally until the drops merge into a continuous stream then no pulses will be generated. The same is true if the fluid reservoir is exhausted. Modern infusion pumps include alarm circuits to detect some of these abnormal conditions but none are foolproof.

Dye dilution computer n=1 c=4,r=3,9

One way to measure cardiac output (in l/min) is to inject a small quantity of dye (usually indocyanine green – ICG) into the venous blood stream close to the heart through a catheter. The dye mixes with the blood, and a sample of arterial blood is drawn off through another catheter and passed through an optical densitometer to detect the concentration of dye. The concentration rises rapidly and then falls. The rate at which blood passes through the heart can be calculated from the area under the curve of concentration and a knowledge of the quantity of dye introduced.

This is an invasive method and the dye is slightly toxic and so it is normally used in conjunction with other invasive procedures during cardiac catheterization in the cardiac catheter laboratory.

The apparatus consists of a high-speed motorized syringe pump, a densitometer sensitive to transmission at 805 nm (for ICG), and a small computer.

Dynamometer n=1 c=1,2

This is a general term for a force or torque meter but is most commonly encountered in medical equipment as a hand dynamometer in the physiotherapy department or physiology research laboratory for exercising the hand and measuring the grip. It may be a simple spring device with a force-indicating pointer, or it may have an electronic sensor and display.

E

Ear mould r=3,4

This is a hollow plastic plug made from an impression of the outer ear and intended to form an almost airtight seal for the coupling tube from a hearing aid to the ear. If an adequate seal is not achieved then there will be a substantial loss of sound amplitude reaching the ear, particularly at lower frequencies. This causes a problem in growing children if the ear mould is not delivered soon after the impression has been taken, and may cause the hearing aid to whistle. An intentional leak (or 'vent') allows the low-frequency sounds to be reduced if this is beneficial to the patient.

Ear moulds may be manufactured in the hospital (audiology department) but more often the impression of the ear is sent to a specialist contractor. To make ear moulds in the hospital the procedure might be to take the outer ear impression using a quick curing (2-5 min) filler. Once set this may be coated with wax from a heated wax bath to slightly enlarge the impression. A plaster of paris cast is then made and this is filled with a liquid which cures to an acrylic polymer. After removal from the plaster it is trimmed and polished, and the sound channel is drilled.

If these processes are undertaken in the hospital department, attention must be given to the health and safety requirements related to the solvents used and machining techniques.

Earth leakage circuit breaker (ELCB) n=50 c=1 r=2

The earth wire in a three wire mains supply is to conduct away any small leakage currents, and also to provide a low resistance path to earth from the case of instrument and cause a fuse to blow if a short circuit should occur inside the equipment. The ELCB monitors the current flowing to earth, usually by measuring the difference between the currents flowing in the live and neutral wires. If this exceeds a preset limit a relay operates to disconnect the supply. The current limit is set to be well above the normal leakage current of the equipment but sufficiently low that the relay can disconnect the supply so quickly that electrocution is avoided.

Since the leakage current is not measured in the earth wire the same principle can be applied to a two-wire supply to a double insulated device. If a fault occurs so that current flows to earth (e.g. through the patient or

85

operator) the supply is disconnected before any harm is done. An ELCB can be incorporated into a mains plug or lead, or may be permanently installed as part of the mains supply. These are coming into very common use now in hospitals and are sometimes called residual current circuit breakers.

Earth leakage current meter/monitor n=3 c=2

Small electric currents leak from equipment driven from the mains electrical supply. These currents are mainly due to capacitance in the supply lead and mains transformer and are usually carried to earth via the protective earth conductor. There are agreed standards (e.g. IEC 601.1/BS 5724) for allowable currents which may flow in the protective earth lead or between other terminals on the equipment (e.g. patient connections and earth) during normal operation, and under single fault conditions.

An earth leakage current monitor is designed to measure these small currents either by insertion into the protective earth path or by connection between the terminals of the equipment and earth. IEC 601.1/BS 5724 requires that the meter indicates combined a.c. and d.c. currents but that frequencies above 1 kHz are de-emphasized by a resistance/capacitance filter with a time constant of 6.7 ms. This is because higher frequencies cause less muscle spasm, and are thus less dangerous.

The allowable earth leakage currents depend on the class and type of the equipment as set out in Table 1.

These current levels are important if they flow inside the body and so clinical equipment is routinely checked for earth leakage and in some special apparatus these currents may be continuously monitored and alarm circuits operated if the levels exceed safe limits. For intermittent testing the supply earth connection is interrupted and an earth leakage current meter inserted into the lead. For continuous monitoring it is usual to detect the difference between the current flowing in the two supply leads, as in the earth leakage circuit breaker (ELCB) commonly used on bench supplies for testing electronic apparatus.

Earth loop tester n=3 c=3

In many countries the mains electricity supply is earth referenced. This produces a live conductor which is at a high voltage (e.g. 240 V) above earth potential, and a neutral, which is actually connected to earth at the local substation. The potential on this lead may be a few volts caused by the ohmic loss between the delivery point and the substation. A third conductor is also provided which is connected to earth within the building. The main purpose of the earth conductor is to carry away the large currents which may flow in the event of the live conductor making electrical connection with the metal

86

Table 1 Allowable leakage currents

	Equipment type		
Current path	Type B	Type BF	Type CF
Earth leakage (mA)	0.5	0.5	0.5
Enclosure to earth (mA)	0.1	0.1	0.01
Patient leakage (mA)	0.1	0.1	0.01

The allowable leakage currents from equipment with a single fault (e.g. broken earth lead) are as in Table 2.

Table 2 Single fault condition: allowable leakage currents

	Equipment type		
Current path	Type B	Type BF	Type CF
Earth leakage (mA)	1.0	1.0	1.0
Enclosure to earth (mA)	0.5	0.5	0.5
Patient leakage (mA)	0.5	0.5	0.05

enclosure of electrical apparatus. The earthing must be of sufficient quality to carry currents well in excess of the fuse capacity to guarantee rapid disconnection of the live supply during faults.

An earth loop tester verifies the integrity of the supply at the substation and within the building by passing a large current (usually 25 A) up the earth lead and back down the neutral lead. This produces a resistance figure for the circuit which will demonstrate whether the earth circuit is capable of blowing the fuses in the live conductor.

Earth loop testers are used by electricians to test the electrical supply installation.

East Radcliffe ventilator $n=5$ $c=4$ $r=2$

An intermittent positive pressure ventilator on which a bellows is opened by a motor and closed by weights, thus regulating the pressure applied to inflate the lungs. It can be used with open or closed anaesthetic circuits and can provide negative pressure during the expiratory phase. It has provision for a humidifier and includes a respirometer.

ECG monitor $n=60$ $c=3,4$ $r=3$

An ECG (electrocardiogram) monitor is a rather loose term applied to cardioscopes, but often wrongly applied to electrocardiographs. For further details see Cardioscope, Arrhythmia detector, Cardiotocograph.

Echocardiograph n=2 c=4,5 r=1

The pattern of movement of structures within the heart can be visualized from the changing echo pattern from ultrasonic waves delivered through the skin above the heart. There are two main types of echocardiograph. The most common type is the M-mode scanner which produces a single line B-scan on a cathode ray tube which shows bright dots corresponding to the various surfaces within the heart. This line of dots is swept slowly across the screen so that the movement of each surface is drawn out showing the waveform of these movements. See M-mode scanner for further details.

Modern echocardiographs may also show a section scan of the heart as seen through a 'window' between the ribs, or from a point on the abdomen below the rib cage. Such scanners are usually sector scanners which provide a triangular image of a part of the heart to show the motion of the chambers and valves. Such devices are used in the cardiology department for investigation of heart valve defects.

There are many types of scanner providing these moving pictures and further details can be found under entries for B-scanner, Section scanner, and Phased array scanner.

Echoencephalograph n=2 c=3,4 r=1

This is an ultrasonic A-scanner used to detect the position of the main membranes within the brain. An ultrasonic transducer applied to the head just above an ear will receive echoes (among others) from the membranes bounding the ventricles and midline (falx cerebri) and the position of these membranes may be displaced if the brain structures are distorted by a tumour, haematoma, or abnormal collection of cerebro-spinal fluid in the ventricles. Echoencephalographs have been used since the 1950s to examine patients with concussion or suspected cranial damage.

The apparatus consists of a transducer, a high-voltage pulse generator, an amplifier to augment the received echoes, and a processing circuit to present the echoes to the cathode ray tube in the form of a base-line indicating distance into the tissue, and vertical deflections corresponding to echo amplitude. Sometimes the apparatus has two transducers so that A-scans are presented simultaneously from each side of the head. The normal symmetry of the brain structures should be presented on each trace in the same positions. Any shift in the positions of the membranes will be immediately obvious.

An automatic midline shift detector has been produced called the 'midliner' which computes any shift without actual presentation of the A-scan.

Edinburgh masker n=2 c=2

Stammering is sometimes exacerbated by the normal mechanism of being able to hear one's own voice. Normal speech production is sometimes achieved if the patient is prevented from hearing his own voice while talking. The Edinburgh masker is designed to do this by a noise being presented to the patient's ears as soon as a microphone (usually in contact with the throat) picks up the sound of the patient's voice. These devices are meant to be worn by patients whenever necessary (rather like hearing aids). They are normally issued on the advice of a speech therapist. A bench model is also available with facility to vary the volume, frequency and characteristics of the masking noise.

Electret microphone

This is a type of electrostatic or capacitor microphone. However, the main feature is that no external polarization voltage is required. This is achieved by the use of a special dielectric medium (electret) between the two plates of the capacitor. These microphones can be extremely small (they are the usual type found in hearing aids) and can have extremely good technical specifications.

Electric response audiometer n=1 c=6 r=3

Although it may be simpler in most cases to test hearing by presenting a sound and asking if it was heard, it is sometimes desirable or necessary to test that the sound has been detected at the cochlea (electrocochleography – ECochG), the brain stem, the cortex (slow vertex response – SVR), or has actuated an auditory reflex (e.g. post auricular muscle response). Apparatus for presenting the stimuli (usually clicks) and detecting the electrical responses are electric response audiometers, and usually contain computer-based signal averagers since the response to a single stimulus might be so small as to be lost in noise.

The need for these tests is where one cannot guarantee that the patient will co-operate fully with conventional audiometry, such as with infants, or with adults who may be exaggerating their symptoms. Also the particular waveforms of the electric responses can assist in diagnosing some of the more obscure conditions.

At present ERA apparatus is only found in special referral centres since there are not large numbers of patients requiring these special tests and there are few staff with the specialized knowledge required for their interpretation. A major expansion in demand may arise in view of the value of the tests in determining hearing loss due to noise exposure at work, and the promise of early diagnosis of deafness in infants.

Electrical impedance cardiac output computer n=1 c=4 r=6

Electrical impedance measurements are used in a number of medical devices, including a type of limb plethysmograph, a skin resistance meter for relaxation control, and a breathing or apnoea monitor. Electrical impedance changes between electrodes at the neck and waist, can relate to the movements of blood. The electrodes take the form of four strips of metal foil, two at the neck and two around the waist. The outer pair of electrodes are fed with a constant electrical current at high frequency (e.g. 100 μA at 100 kHz) and the inner pair are connected to an amplifier and phase sensitive detector, and any necessary computing apparatus.

Experimental work suggests good accuracy of cardiac output calculation by this method as compared to dye dilution, and Fick methods. However, the devices have not gained wide acceptance.

Electrical stimulator n=15 c=2,3 r=3,4

Nerves and muscles in the body produce electric potentials when they operate, and conversely they can be made to operate by electrical stimulation. Electrical stimulators are widely used in hospitals.

In the physiotherapy department stimulators exist which may provide direct, alternating, pulsating, or pulsed waveforms, and are used to exercise the muscles by stimulation through electrodes placed on the skin. The apparatus required for this is often called a Faradic treatment unit, or electrotherapy set.

Electrical stimulators are also sometimes used by anaesthetists during surgery to demonstrate the muscular response to stimulation of a nerve (usually applied to the arm or wrist via electrodes on the skin). Muscle relaxants used during surgery should abolish the response.

Stimulators exist now which are used for the relief of pain. These transcutaneous electrical neural stimulators (TENS) appear to suppress other pains in the same general area where the stimulation is applied. Electrical stimulation of trigger points is also claimed to be effective. Known trigger points (from acupuncture) are said to display lower skin resistance than other sites. The use of TENS at these points may produce therapeutic effects remote from the sites in question. The mechanism by which these effects are produced is poorly understood. The same can be said of electroanaesthesia and electrosleep.

Electrical stimulators are also used in the neurology department for diagnostic tests on the nervous system. A common test measures nerve conduction velocity using stimulation via skin electrodes but stimulation may also be applied directly to nerve trunks or into the brain during specialized procedures, but these are less common.

Cardiac pacemakers are electrical stimulators which apply short pulses at the desired heart rate to a site within the heart. These pulses are intended to trigger (prompt) the natural pacemaking mechanisms of the heart and may be required for a short period (in which case an external stimulator may be used with a long wire leading to the heart) or they may be implantable devices remaining in for a number of years before new batteries need fitting.

Other types of stimulator exist including those used to cause contraction of leg or arm muscles as an aid to rehabilitation after spinal injuries, injury to peripheral nerves or muscles, and those stimulators intended for use on the muscles of the pelvic floor as a treatment for incontinence. Electrodes for such devices may be implanted, indwelling, transcutaneous (needles), or surface.

Electrical stimulators may have controls to set the pulse length, pulse repetition frequency, pulse amplitude, and triggering modes. Modern stimulators should either be battery operated or fully electrically isolated.

Electro-aerometer $n=1$ $c=3$

This is designed for accurate measurement of airflow during speech, and is intended for research applications in phonetics, linguistics, and psychology and may be used in the hospital speech therapy department. It employs two airflow transducers (anemometers) which register separately inflow and outflow of air through the nose and mouth. Each transducer unit consists of a specially designed rubber valve in which the aperture is registered by means of a light beam transmitted through the valve and detected by a photo-diode. The transducers are connected to two d.c. amplifiers and there is also a microphone amplifier and a 10 ms integrating filter. Air flow rates up to about 60 l/min are catered for. The system works through a standard anaesthetic mask.

Electroanaesthesia apparatus $n=0$ $c=2$ $r=4$

Something resembling the state of chemically induced anaesthesia may be achieved by passing pulsed electrical currents of 5–50 mA through the head for several minutes. This is similar to electrosleep treatment but employs currents 10 to 100 times greater. The mechanism of operation is poorly understood and is little used.

The apparatus for electroanaesthesia is a conventional electrical stimulator with controls to vary the pulse rate, pulse width, and voltage or current. The current is normally passed through the head between the frontal and occipital locations employing large area electrodes usually covered with saline-soaked gauze sponges.

Electroanalgesia apparatus n=5 c=2 r=4

Electrical stimulation of tissue has been shown to be effective in the reduction of pain in some disorders. The most common clinical use of this is transcutaneous electrical neural stimulation (TENS) in which pulsed stimulation is provided for long periods using large area electrodes over the site of the pain. The stimulation causes a tingling sensation and also reduces the level of the perceived pain. About one third of patients with chronic pain benefit from this treatment which may be applied in the case of herniated discs, injury, arthritis, strain, and postoperative pain. Typical stimulation parameters are 100–150 pulses/s, pulse width of 250–400 μs, and output levels of 20–35 mA. Such devices may be used by the patient at home, with parameters and treatment periods set according to the daily needs of the patient. Treatment periods may extend for several hours at a time, and the relief from pain may persist for an equivalent period.

Electroanalgesia may also be applied by direct stimulation to the nerves or spinal cord. Although this may be less applicable to a large population suffering from chronic pain it may be used in selected patients employing needle electrodes or implanted electrodes and receivers, the power source being external to the body with an inductive loop operating at a frequency of 100–500 kHz.

Electrocardiograph n=30 c=3,4 r=3,9

Electrical signals arising from the heart can be picked up through skin electrodes and presented on a relatively slow-moving chart as the electrocardiogram (ECG). The origin of each part of the ECG waveform is very well understood and electrocardiographic records now represent one of the commonest measurement procedures performed on patients in hospital. Abnormalities in the waveform are indicative of various types of heart disease and of cardiac distress arising from other illnesses or biochemical disturbances.

Electrocardiograms are performed in the cardiac department, and also in the wards of the hospital. The electrocardiogram is also monitored on CRT (cardioscope) screens in many wards, and in the operating theatre, but not always for the purpose of making diagnoses, more the monitoring of the condition of the patient as reflected by the strength and rate of the signals.

An electrocardiograph consists of a set of electrodes and leads which are placed on the body according to a conventional plan. The most commonly used of these electrodes are placed on the legs and arms, and others are placed in a line roughly over the heart. The electrocardiograph has a lead selector switch to configure these electrodes into different groupings to produce differential signals which represent different planes through the heart. The waveform seen at each of the switch positions is slightly different.

Electrocardiographs are normally portable or mounted on light trolleys so that they can be moved around the hospital, and are often battery operated. The most common instruments record one lead configuration at a time, although three-channel versions are becoming common. The ECG signal is normally about 1 mV in amplitude, and with frequency components from less than 1 Hz to 100 Hz. These are amplified in a differential amplifier having a frequency response of typically 0.02 to 100 Hz, and very high common-mode rejection ratio (CMRR) to cut down the a.c. interference picked up from the mains supply by the long electrode leads. A standard paper speed of 25 mm/s and sensitivity of 10 mm/mV is used for most recordings and the amplitudes of the various parts of the waveform are usually quoted in millimetres.

A typical ECG recording procedure would consist of cleaning the skin, abrading, attaching electrodes and applying the conductive electrode jelly, and with the patient relaxed, recording a few centimetres of the ECG at each of the standard lead positions. These are then sent for diagnostic reporting by a cardiac physician. The foetal ECG signal is also sometimes monitored during pregnancy and labour to record the foetal heart rate.

Electrocautery apparatus n=10 c=3,4 r=4

This is the application of a hot probe or wire for cutting tissue or for coagulating and sterilizing it. The apparatus normally consists of a low-voltage high-current source applied to a probe through a flexible lead. This technique is also covered under cautery apparatus.

Electrocochleograph r=3

The apparatus on which one would record the electrocochleograph (ECochG) would most likely be an electric response audiometer consisting of a calibrated click or tone generator and earpiece, and an amplifier and signal averager connected to a needle electrode which is passed (usually under general or local anaesthetic) through the eardrum so that its tip lies on the promontory of the cochlea. There is an electrical response to each click which is dependent on the amplitude of the sound stimulus. Such apparatus is usually found in the audiology department.

Electroconvulsive therapy apparatus n=3 c=3 r=4

The treatment of some anxiety states and schizophrenia may include the passage of large electrical currents (1 A or more) through the head in short pulses (100–500 ms) often at the mains supply frequency.

Such equipment is found in the psychiatry department.

Electrode r=3,4,6,9

To record the ECG, EEG, EMG, etc. electrodes must be used as transducers to convert an ionic flow of current in the body to an electronic flow along a wire. These are usually made of metal. Two important characteristics of electrodes are electrode potential and contact impedance. Good electrodes will have low stable figures for both of the above characteristics.

Electrode potential arises because a metal electrode in contact with an electrolyte (body fluids) forms a half cell with a potential dependent upon the metal in use and the ions in the electrolyte. One might expect that two electrodes of the same material would produce the same electrode potential which would cancel out in any recording, but the actual potentials do depend upon the conditions of contact; for instance, if two steel electrodes are placed in contact with the skin there may be a net contact potential between them of 100 mV. This might cause serious problems when amplifying signals in the microvolt region.

The most widely used electrodes for biomedical applications are silver electrodes which have been coated with silver chloride by electrolysing them for a short time in a sodium chloride solution. When chlorided the surface is black and has a very large surface area. A pair of such electrodes might have a combined electrode potential below 5 mV.

All electrodes suffer from variations in contact resistance due to movement, and the drying out of any coupling medium. This is improved by setting the electrode back slightly from the surface of the skin (floating electrode) on a quantity of coupling jelly (electrolyte paste). A further problem may arise if there is any direct current flowing through the electrode arising from faulty equipment or from small (microamp) bias currents in the measuring amplifier circuit. Over a period of time these currents cause chemical changes at the surface of the electrode causing polarization with consequent increase in the electrode potential. This may cause drift of the electrode potential and damage to the skin due to the chemical action. Many types of recording electrodes exist including metal discs, needles, suction electrodes, glass microelectrodes, foetal scalp clips or screws, etc.

Electrodes are also used to inject electricity into the body as in faradism, TENS, surgical diathermy and physiotherapy diathermy. Electrodes also exist in some analytical apparatus to measure the concentration of specific ions.

Electroencephalograph (EEG) n=3 c=5,6 r=3,9

Electrical signals from the brain can be picked up by electrodes attached to the scalp. Differential signals between electrodes over different parts of the brain, and monopolar signals between each electrode and a reference, typically give signal amplitudes of between 10 and 300 μV, with frequency content between 0.5 and 40 Hz. The apparatus normally produces a wide paper strip with eight or sixteen simultaneous tracings showing the patterns derived from electrodes placed over different parts of the brain, and the relationship between these. Computer analysis of electroencephalograms is possible, but in most everyday use the paper strip is read directly by a technician or neurologist.

These machines are found in the neurology department or in a special sub-section of this called the EEG department. Patients are referred for investigation of suspected abnormalities of the brain which may arise from disease, injury, or may be congenital in origin (e.g. epilepsy). There are standard electrode configurations and standard procedures for the test, since the EEG may change considerably even with the mood of the patient. In some tests a stimulus is applied such as a flashing light. Evoked response averaging of the EEG is sometimes applied to identify which part of the EEG waveform relates to a particular stimulus, but is more often performed on dedicated machinery in the departments which use the results (e.g. electric response audiometry in the audiology department).

A typical EEG machine would consist of a head harness to hold the electrodes, a set of electrodes and leads, an input selector box with switches to group the electrodes into the standard configurations, preamplifiers with variable settings and time-constant switch to define the low-frequency cut-off, and filters for high-frequency cut-off. There would also be a calibrating facility. Following the preamplifiers are the pen-drive amplifiers, with shift and ink controls. The actual writing mechanism may be pen and ink, or it may be an ink spray type, in which ink is sprayed on to the paper from a jet mounted on a galvanometer a few centimetres from the paper. This type has the advantage of a very high frequency response. Photographic type recorders are possible, but unusual.

A one or two channel version is sometimes used as a 'cerebral function monitor' in intensive care or in the operating theatre. This produces a slow-moving paper chart record of the EEG on which the amplitude is taken to indicate the state of the patient. The waveform of the EEG is completely ignored. Since clinical death is commonly defined from the absence of an

EEG, these devices have a use which is quite distinct from the diagnostic uses in the EEG department.

Electroglottograph n=1 c=2,3

Also called a laryngograph this produces a display on a cathode ray tube representing movements of the vocal cords. The signal is derived from ECG-type electrodes placed each side of the glottis, which measure electrical impedance changes. Such devices are used in the speech therapy department to aid diagnosis of voice disorders and are used in a form of feedback therapy to help the patient make sounds correctly. The voiscope is an extended version of the electroglottograph displaying speech fundamental frequency.

Electrogustometer n=1 c=2

Also known as a 'taste tester' or gustometer, this device is an electrical stimulator for measuring the threshold of taste by the passage of a small d.c. current from one side of the tongue to either the tip of the tongue or another midline point on the cranium (e.g. nose). The threshold current should be approximately equal on both sides of the tongue. A significant inequality may be suggestive of a lesion affecting the fifth cranial (trigeminal) nerve. Electrogustometers are sometimes used in neurophysiology or ENT departments for differential diagnosis in Bell's palsy.

Electrolysis unit n=2 c=1,2

Direct electric current passing through the body causes chemical changes due to electrolysis of the salts. The effect can be used to destroy tissue selectively for the removal of hair and small skin blemishes. In these cases a large positive electrode is placed on the skin to provide a return path for the current and a negative electrode (cathode) with a small tip is applied to the point being treated. Such units may be called electrolysis or catholysis units.

Electromagnetic blood flowmeter n=1 c=5 r=3,9

Faraday's principle of electromagnetic induction can be applied to any electrical conductor (including blood) which moves through a magnetic field. The electromagnetic blood flowmeter is sometimes used during vascular surgery to measure the quantity of blood passing through a vessel or graft, before during or after surgery. A circular probe with a gap to fit the vessel is fitted around the vessel. This probe applies an alternating magnetic field across the vessel and detects the voltage induced by the flow via small electrodes in contact with the vessel.

Alternating magnetic fields (typically at 400 Hz) are used since the induced voltages are in the microvolt region and d.c. electrode potentials may cause significant errors with unchanging magnetic fields. A number of probes are required to fit the various diameters of blood vessel.

An alternative design carries the sensing device on the tip of a special catheter which passes inside the vessel and generates a magnetic field in the space around it and has the electrodes on its surface.

Electromagnetic flowmeters have existed for measurement of blood flow rate outside the body during open heart surgery.

Electromyograph (EMG) n=3 c=4,5 r=3

Electrical activity of nerves and muscles can be measured to demonstrate abnormalities of the neuromuscular system arising from disease or injury. The action of nerves and muscle is essentially electrical by which information is transmitted along nerves as a series of electrical discharges carrying information in the pulse repetition frequency, which may be in the range of 1 to 100 pulses/s. Contraction of muscle fibres is also associated with an electrical discharge which can be detected by measuring electrodes or brought about by electrical stimulation.

Most electromyography is performed using needle electrodes, normally in the form of hollow needles with one or more wires down the centre appearing as small electrodes at the tip. These needles can be placed within nerve trunks, or muscles to record the discharges arising from a number of fibres close to the tip. Such electrodes may detect signals up to about 500 μV with frequency content extending from 10 Hz to 5 kHz. Since these frequencies are in the audible range, it is common to present them through a loudspeaker after amplification. The sound of the EMG assists the operator to position the electrodes and to study the effects of various manoeuvres, such as voluntary contraction of muscle.

Many EMG tests involve the use of stimulators to induce discharges in a nerve trunk, and detect the response by surface electrodes over a muscle served by that nerve. In this case the signals may be as large as 2 mV, and may be presented audibly or for recording on a high-speed chart recorder. Such evoked response tests might be for determining the nerve conduction time, or for assessing the performance of the neuromuscular control system. There are many different disorders of the nervous system and EMG examination has to be tailored to the particular requirements of the individual patient. Thus, these tests are normally carried out by a specialist in electromyography in the neurology department.

EMG equipment consists of recording electrodes, preamplifiers, which are normally placed very close to the patient to avoid pick-up of electrical interference, amplifiers to provide the correct gain, calibration and frequency characteristics, a display system (usually a CRT), a range of integrators and averagers partly to achieve some data compression (chart records may be very long and difficult to read), and a recording medium, which is often a photographic (fibre-optic) system.

Electronarcosis apparatus n=0 c=2 r=4

This term is used to describe any phenomenon induced as a result of the passage of electric currents through the head and may extend from electrosleep employing very low currents (e.g. 500 μA average) to electro-convulsive therapy employing currents of 1 A or more for a fraction of a second.

Except for electro-convulsive therapy (ECT) such techniques are not used routinely in hospitals. The generators for electronarcosis are pulse generators with variable pulse rate, pulse width, and output voltage or current.

Electronystagmograph (ENG) n=2 c=4

Nystagmus is an involuntary eye movement which occurs during an attack of dizziness or vertigo. The electronystagmograph can be used to record spontaneous or induced nystagmus by placing surface electrodes (usually EEG-type silver/silver chloride fluid column electrodes) at either side of the patient's eyes. The small voltages so recorded are derived from the corneo–retinal potential of the eyeball. The electronystagmograph consists of an amplifier with filters (typically 0.1 Hz to 30 Hz) connected to a chart recorder with a paper speed of 1 cm/s. Single channel machines are most common and record the lateral eye movement of both eyes although multichannel machines allow the separate analysis of each eye in horizontal and vertical planes. This is sometimes called an electro-oculograph (EOG).

Electronystagmographs are normally found in audiology departments and are used in conjunction with caloric apparatus and an optokinetic drum to induce nystagmus. Many of the tests are conducted in total darkness since the patient's observed environment has a large effect upon his eye movements (nystagmus usually disappears if the patient is able to fix his gaze on something he can see). The infrared viewer and Frenzel glasses are other devices to enable eye movement to be assessed without the patient being able to fix his gaze.

Electro-oculograph n=2 c=5 r=9

There is a steady d.c. potential between the cornea and retina of the eye. Electrodes placed on the skin each side of the eye record a zero voltage when the gaze is straight ahead but a negative or positive voltage as the eye moves to the left and right of this position. There is an almost linear relationship between the horizontal angle of the gaze and the voltage produced. The recording of this voltage is called the electro-oculogram (EOG). Electrodes may also be placed above and below the eye to record vertical movements.

The electro-oculograph is commonly used for recording eye movements in sleep and dream movements and also for recording nystagmus, which is the involuntary eye movement which occurs during dizziness or vertigo. The EOG is also used in the eye clinic or electrophysiology laboratory for assessing the strength of the corneo–retinal potential during changes in ambient light conditions. Some disorders of the retina exhibit abnormal or absent changes in the corneo–retinal potential during dark and light adaptation processes. For these tests the patient is asked to move his eyes to focus on two fixation lights 15 degrees either side of centre to produce alternating voltages which are dependent on the corneo–retinal potential. As the ambient light conditions are changed the voltage will change producing a graph of this change on the electro-oculograph.

The instrument for this employs silver–silver chloride electrodes each side of the eyes and two recording amplifiers with frequency response from d.c. to 50 Hz. The potentials detected may vary from 0.05 to 3.5 mV. The recording system may be integrated with a generalized electrophysiology set used for recording the ERG, VEP/VER, the EMG, and possibly the EEG. The patient may be given verbal instructions to look at the fixation lights or the lights may flash alternately. Red fixation lights are normally used since these do not affect the dark adaptation process.

Electrophoresis apparatus n=5 c=3 r=9

The apparatus consists basically of a high voltage (e.g. 250 V) d.c. generator which causes a small current (4–6 mA) to flow along a paper or cellulose acetate strip linking two baths of buffer solution. Samples of body fluids are introduced on to the strip and individual components (proteins, enzymes, and antibodies) move at different rates along the strip under the influence of the electric currents. After a time the process is arrested and the strip is fixed and stained for examination under a densitometer which produces a graph of optical density identifying the concentration of the particular components.

Electroretinograph n=1 c=5 r=9

When the retina of the eye is stimulated by a flash of light, there is a characteristic sequence of electrical potentials generated within the retina. The clinical electroretinogram (ERG) is a recording of these potentials as detected between an electrode on or close to the cornea and an indifferent electrode placed on the forehead, cheek or ear lobe. The corneal electrode may be in the form of a contact lens with a steel or silver wire embedded in the inner surface, or it may be a piece of gold leaf tucked under the lower lid close to the cornea. A skin electrode on the lower lid of the eye can be used instead of the corneal electrodes but the result is less satisfactory.

It is common to perform the test with the eyes 'dark adapted', that is after spending several minutes in complete darkness. Under these conditions the ERG response is relatively large (e.g. 200 μV) and produces a wave with several distinct components covering about two seconds, but the components used for clinical diagnosis (known as A and B-waves) occur in the first half second.

The flash of light is normally provided from a stroboscopic flash unit and it is repeated a number of times so that the resulting electrical response can be fed to a signal averager to improve the signal-to-noise ratio and to reduce artefacts such as the blink response. Thus the recording apparatus will include a preamplifier capable of dealing with input signals between 0 and 1 mV, with frequency response from 0 to 50 Hz (true d.c. response is not in fact required), a signal averager, and a display or recording device.

The ERG apparatus is normally found in the eye clinic or electrophysiological laboratory or it is part of a generalized instrument which may also be used for the electro-oculogram (EOG), electromyogram (EMG), possibly the visual evoked response (VER), and the electroencephalogram (EEG). The ERG is commonly used to assist in making a diagnosis of the various inherited disorders of the eye.

Electrosleep apparatus n=0 c=2 r=4

Electrosleep, or electronarcosis, which is a more general term for the passage of electric currents through the head, may be used to induce sleep and for the treatment of insomnia, anxiety, depression and irritability. There are also reports of its use for the treatment of chronic alcoholism, hypertension, hypothalamic disorders and peptic ulcers.

The general principle is to deliver small currents (time averaged to about 500 μA) for one hour or more. The electrodes may be saline-gauze sponges over metal plates applied between frontal and occipital locations.

The mechanism of operation is not properly understood and such techniques are not used routinely in most hospitals.

Electrosurgery unit n=14 c=4 r=3,4

This is a surgical diathermy apparatus. Most surgical operations utilize electrosurgery to create a bloodless entry into the body, to treat or remove lesions from inside the body, to remove unwanted hair and to control bleeding. An electrosurgery unit provides a high power (50-400 W) source of

100

high-frequency alternating current at between 0.5 and 3 MHz. The unit may also provide current for endoscopy lamps and for electrocautery.

The apparatus may be unipolar, delivering current between a small active electrode and a large indifferent (or dispersive) electrode, or it may be bipolar in which case the current is delivered between the two arms of a special forceps with insulated handles. There are two main functions, cutting and coagulating. In the case of cutting, a continuous sinusoidal current is delivered to a pointed or sharp electrode to yield clean cutting as the cellular water is rapidly volatized at the point of contact with the probe (active electrode). In coagulation a larger active electrode (e.g. ball-tipped) provides short pulses of high voltage which cause desiccation and fulguration of tissue by an electric arc which coagulates the tissue and arrests blood flow.

Diathermy is not a proper description for the technique, since little heat is generated within the bulk of the tissue between the two electrodes; most is generated at the point of contact between the active electrode and the tissues being treated. The waveform is important in providing current suitable for cutting or coagulating, but these may be blended to provide power suitable for both. More important is the shape of the active electrode.

Modern electrosurgery machines have transistor current generators, but many valve (tube) types are in use, some with spark-gap generators. Transistor circuits have shown difficulty in the past in generating the high voltages required for coagulation. With unipolar electrosurgery the indifferent plate used to be connected to earth. This created a risk of electrocution by earthing the patient, and so later types were not earthed but included a ground reference capacitor which limited the path to earth for low-frequency (e.g. 50 Hz) currents. There is still a risk of diathermy burns with ground referenced systems if the indifferent electrode is poorly fitted or disconnected. Later types are earth free except for a route provided by stray capacitance between the machine, the patient, and earth. These types often include a sensing circuit to recognize detrimental changes in the earth reference arrangement.

Special loop electrodes are also used, particularly during intra-cavity surgery, such as prostatectomy, endoscopic electrosurgery in the rectum, vagina or abdominal cavity, which can be used to cut conical sections from diseased tissue.

Electrotherapy apparatus n=10 c=4 r=10

Electrotherapy is a form of physiotherapy in which muscles are stimulated directly or indirectly via the nerves to exercise denervated or partially denervated muscles, or to develop wasted muscles after immobilization, and to develop the blood supply. The most common form of treatment is to apply saline or conductive gel-covered electrodes directly over the sites to be stimulated. Variations on this may include placing the whole limb in a bath in which the electrodes are placed, or by the use of internal electrodes in the vagina or rectum for developing the pelvic floor muscles.

Current waveforms may be interrupted direct current, sinusoidal low-frequency currents (e.g. 50 Hz), or faradic currents. Faradic currents are bursts of short pulses such as can be generated from induction coils or latterly using electronic generators. An electrotherapy apparatus may be a multi-purpose generator and electrode set for delivering a selection of these different treatment modes, and varying the intensity, pulse lengths, and providing particular treatment regimes employing bursts of pulses or sinusoidal current, steadily rising currents and with variable periods of rest between each muscle contraction. The physiotherapist plans a treatment regime for each patient and decides on the siting of electrodes and type of current to be used.

The patient electrodes are normally isolated from the mains supply and earth.

Therapeutic diathermy apparatus used in the physiotherapy department employing high-frequency currents (usually 27 MHz) is sometimes termed electrotherapy apparatus. These short-wave diathermy machines, and also microwave diathermy machines do induce electric currents into the body but do not stimulate muscles. The principal effect is to generate heat deep within the tissue to stimulate the blood supply and reduce inflammation.

Elephant tubing r=2

This is a name commonly given to large-bore corrugated breathing tubes used on anaesthetic apparatus.

Emerson cuirass ventilator r=4

This applies a negative pressure around the thorax (rather than over the whole body as in the case of the 'iron lung') which may be used to enhance ventilation of the lungs.

EMI scanner

This is an early name for what is now known as a CT scanner. The name derives from the company (EMI) which produced the first CT scanner.

Emission spectroscope n=1 c=4 r=9

In medical work this is mainly used to calculate the molar fraction of nitrogen in a gas mixture. It is used in some lung function tests.

A tiny quantity of the gas mixture to be sampled is drawn through a needle valve by a high vacuum pump to provide pressures of 1 to 4 mmHg and this gas mixture is ionized between two electrodes in an ionization chamber. The gases emit light which is detected by a phototube after passing though an optical filter to remove wavelengths outside the range of 310–480 nm. An amplifier and linearizing circuit is connected to the phototube to produce a figure for nitrogen concentration. Nitrogen concentration from 0 to 80% can be measured with considerable accuracy with response time of the order of 40 ms. Oxygen and carbon dioxide do not interfere with the accuracy. However, helium and argon can produce errors.

Emission tomography (ECAT) scanner n=1 c=8

A variation on the general idea employed in the CT scanner employs radioactive sources within the body. Radiopharmaceuticals are taken up selectively by different tissues, and an ECAT scanner can be used to create an image of their distribution in a single plane (section) by rotating a gamma camera around the body. The image of radionuclide distribution is assembled by computer. Such scanners are relatively new additions to the possible imaging techniques in the nuclear medicine department.

Endobronchial tube c=1 r=2

Anaesthesia or assisted ventilation during procedures in which access to the lung is required may be performed via a catheter fed into a bronchus so that not all the lung is being ventilated. An endobronchial tube can be passed into a section of the lung and an airtight seal created by the inflation of one or more cuffs, often covered with a nylon mesh to provide a rough surface to prevent dislodging. Types available include the Robertshaw twin lumen, Gordon Green R, the Vernon Thompson bronchus blocker, and Brompton triple cuff. This latter has a spare cuff in case of puncture during the procedure.

Endoradiosonde

This is a radio transmitter operating from inside the body. The best known example is the radio pill which is a small transmitter which can be swallowed to record electrical, pressure or pH changes within the gut. Similar devices can be introduced into the bladder to record pressure changes. They are usually epoxy encapsulated and contain a simple Hartley oscillator circuit operating at low frequency (e.g. 0.5 MHz) which is detected outside the body with a loop aerial. More complex devices are possible which may be implanted but these are not used clinically.

Endoscope n=30 c=3,4 r=4

Direct visualization of a diseased area inside the body can be achieved by using a telescope or tube passed through a natural orifice or through a small incision in the skin. This may be rigid employing a series of lenses, or flexible employing optic fibres to convey the illuminating light, and to convey the image to the eyepiece. The endoscope is often fitted with one or more extra channels through which operating instruments may be passed such as electrosurgery probes, or manipulating, grasping or crushing forceps. These channels may also be used for delivering fluids or gas, providing suction, or passing sampling catheters or laser light pipes. In the case of flexible endoscopes the operating handle may also include controls for manipulating the tip to the site required.

There is almost no part of the body not now accessible for endoscopes for viewing or treatment, and typical sites include the ear, throat, urinary tract, lungs, intestines and abdominal cavity.

In the case of the sigmoidoscope used for examining the rectum and sigmoid colon the scope may consist of a hollow cylinder without special optics.

Endotracheal connector n=200 c=1 r=2

During anaesthesia, this is used to join the endotracheal tube to the catheter mount and essentially consists of a small bent tube of metal or plastic. These may be a single piece (e.g. Rowbottom, Magill, Cobb's, Rink's Cardiff) or two part (e.g. Nosworthy, Knight's paediatric, BOC international 15), allowing easy disconnection for bronchial suction or circuit change. On single part connectors a stoppered suction port may be provided. Special types are also available for connecting to nasal endotracheal tubes and for procedures in which the patient's neck is bent some way from the usual position.

Endotracheal tube c=1 r=2

During anaesthesia it is common to deliver the gases and vapours, and provide assisted ventilation via a tube in the trachea. If positive pressure ventilation is used then an airtight seal is required, and this is usually effected by an inflatable cuff near the end of the tube. The tubes may be rubber or plastic, have an internal diameter of 8–11 mm (for adults), include a valve mechanism to control inflation and deflation of the cuff, a balloon at the distal end of the inflation mechanism to indicate whether the endotracheal balloon is inflated, and a suitable shape to sit easily in the pharynx or nasopharynx without straining the connector or seal in the trachea.

Types exist for passage via the nose or mouth and particular designs exist to prevent kinking, end occlusion by the tracheal wall, and to suit particular procedures. Examples of common and special tubes are plain and cuffed Magill, Magill flexo-metallic paediatric, Cole neonatal, Riplex neonatal resuscitation, Enderby paediatric tube, Oxford non-kinking, and the Jackson Rees paediatric tube (which includes its own T-piece and suction facility).

Entonox apparatus n=50 c=3 r=2

This is a system of valves and pressure regulators which fit on to a cylinder or pipe terminal of Entonox (50/50 nitrous oxide and oxygen) to provide intermittent (demand) flow of analgesia gases for use in labour, emergency surgery and dental surgery. Since Entonox does not liquefy under pressure the cylinder need not be kept upright in use, and the pressure gauge gives a true indication of cylinder contents, but if stored below zero centigrade the gases separate and must be warmed and agitated before use.

Enzyme analyser

This is also called a reaction rate analyser and usually works as a centrifugal analyser. Samples of body fluids are diluted and pipetted into cuvettes arranged around the outside of a centrifuge rotor. As the rotor starts to spin, reagents are drawn down into the cuvettes and a reaction begun which changes the colour or optical density of the samples in the cuvettes. The light from a colorimeter or densitometer passes through each of the cuvettes in turn so that the progress of the reaction in each cuvette is monitored throughout the reaction. The reaction rate (corresponding to the concentration of particular enzymes) can be assessed from the rate of change at the start of the reaction, or half way through. See also Reaction rate analyser.

It is also possible to measure some enzyme reaction rates using a continuous flow or discrete sample analyser.

Epilation unit n=1 c=2

For removal of hairs, usually by electrolysis (catholysis), a fine metal probe is brought into contact with the base of a hair and a direct electrical current is passed through. Chemical changes caused by the current in the vicinity of the probe tip cause the hair follicle to die. The probe forms the negative electrode (cathode) and the positive electrode is attached to the skin nearby. The positive electrode has a large surface area so that the current density beneath it never reaches toxic levels. The same instrument may sometimes be called an electrolysis unit, catholysis unit, or depilator.

Ergometric recording system n=1 c=5,6

Patients with heart disease may undergo changes in the ECG along with blood pressure changes during exercise. Exercise may be undertaken and measured using a treadmill or a bicycle type of ergonometer. The patient exercises on the ergonometer and measurements are made of the work output, ECG and blood pressure. The system may have alarms for specific changes in the ECG or blood pressure.

Evoked response averager n=5 c=4 r=3,9

Although this has a common meaning, in medical equipment it normally refers to an electrical signal averager of the type used for averaging the response to a stimulus (electrical, light, sound, or the use of a short-acting drug). The response being monitored may be the heart rate, EEG, EMG, blood pressure, etc. and these may undergo fluctuations due to external interference or natural variations. If the response evoked by the stimulus is likely to be small compared with these other fluctuations, signal averaging may be employed to demonstrate the effect of the stimulus alone.

The usual method is to repeat the test a number of times and add up all the responses so that natural fluctuations cancel out since they are not linked to the time of the stimulus. For evoked response averaging applied to an optical or auditory stimulus affecting the EEG the test may be repeated a large number of times in rapid succession so that a very small response may be detected in the presence of quite substantial noise. For a drug test, which may be carried out once only on each of a number of patients, the number of tests may be small.

Averagers are commonly found in the EEG, EMG and audiology clinics of hospitals and are usually microcomputers which hold the results in a computer memory so that each new result is added to the previous one in the computer memory. Tests performed using evoked response averagers include electric response audiometry (ERA), visual evoked response (VER), and electroretinogram (ERG).

Exeter lip sensor n=1 c=2

This is a training aid for patients requiring a lip-seal reminder. It consists of a lip electrode which hooks on to the lower lip connected to an electronic control unit having a buzzer which sounds continuously when the lips are open. Such devices may be used by speech therapists.

Exeter visual speech aid n=1 c=2,3

This is a device to assist in the treatment of poor soft palate movement. An intra-oral appliance is made by a dental surgeon and when connected to the electronic control unit it may be used as part of a training programme to produce co-ordinated movement of the soft palate. Such devices might be used by speech therapists.

Expiratory valve n=200 c=1 r=2

Often called just the 'pop-off', 'relief', or 'spill' valve, which can be fixed or adjustable, this is used in an anaesthetic breathing circuit to allow the expired gases and other excess gases to vent to atmosphere (usually) and then to prevent outside air from entering the breathing circuit. The most commonly used type is the Heidbrink valve or modifications of this. It is usually in a wide bore T-piece which fits in line with the breathing tube and usually as close to the patient as possible. The side arm of the T-piece contains a simple valve in the form of a light disc held against a ring by a spring. The spring tension can be adjusted by screwing the valve top. As the top is screwed in the pressure required to lift the disc becomes greater until the valve is locked in the off position with the top screwed right down. Locking the valve is useful for controlled or assisted ventilation.

If the valve opening pressure is too high there will be significant resistance to expiration. On the other hand it must not be so low that the reservoir bag will empty spontanteously. Some types include a calibrated valve spring adjuster (e.g. Magill, McKesson).

Adjustable valves are used during several types of inhalation anaesthesia: spontaneous breathing, assisted, and manually controlled ventilation. In mechanically controlled ventilation the valve is shut and gases are vented through the attached ventilator. Alternative valve designs may control exit pressure by varying the weight of the ball, by varying a magnetically controlled disc, by varying a movable piston or by varying the valve orifice.

Eye magnet n=2 c=3

A very powerful electromagnet with a pointed applicator is used to extract small metal fragments from the eye. It is brought close to the eye and the power turned on by a foot switch. Considerable heat is generated by these units and so some care is needed to avoid prolonged use or application to the skin or dressings. They are operated from the mains electricity supply.

F

Face mask r=2

This is more properly called the facepiece, as used to deliver gases during some anaesthesia and resuscitation procedures.

Facepiece n=200 c=1 r=2

This is the facemask used to induce anaesthesia and for resuscitation procedures. It is normally designed to fit the face (nose, or nose and mouth) to provide an airtight seal. The mask consists of a mount (with connection for the breathing circuit), body, and an edge. The edge must seal on to the face without the need for excessive pressure. This is achieved either by flaps, a flexible edge with stiffening, or by inflation of an air filled cuff/cushion around the edge. If the edge is inflatable there is usually a small valve protruding through which air can be injected or withdrawn to change the fit. The pressure required is low and it can be inflated by mouth.

It is difficult to fit every face and so it is usual for a range of different sizes to be available.

Faraday cage r=3

For the measurement of very small electrical signals (such as EEG or EMG) in environments with high levels of electrostatic noise it is sometimes desirable to make a whole room which is impervious to electrostatic fields. This can be achieved by including a metal mesh in the doors, walls, ceiling, floor and (if they must be present) the windows. All of the mesh must be connected together and connected to earth. Although this technique has been used widely in the past, modern equipment can be made with very high common mode rejection ratio (CMRR, e.g. 120 dB) which makes such arrangements unnecessary except in the noisiest environments such as next to an elevator shaft.

Unfortunately such cages have little effect on the penetration of magnetic fields.

Faradic treatment unit n=5 c=3,4 r=10

Direct electrical stimulation of the nerves and muscles as a form of

108

physiotherapy may be delivered through surface electrodes or in a current bath. The current may be pulses of direct current up to 3 seconds in length, bursts of low-frequency alternating current (typically 50 Hz), or series of short pulses a few milliseconds in length. This latter form of treatment is called faradism (the name derives from the generation of short pulses from faradic coils in which an inductor generates short pulses when its current supply is interrupted).

Faradic treatment units may be used for the activation of denervated or partially denervated muscles for the toning of wasted muscles, and for developing the blood supply in wasted limbs. The faradic treatment unit usually allows variation of the pulse length, height, and control over a range of pulsating wave forms including slowly rising pulse heights with periods of rest between them to allow the muscles to recover. Modern units are electronic but earlier units employ an induction coil such as the Smart Bristow faradic coil.

Although saline-soaked electrodes are normally applied over the muscles to be stimulated, the whole limb may be placed in a bath containing the electrodes (current bath), or an internal electrode may be used such as those used for the treatment of stress incontinence which employ vaginal or rectal electrodes in an attempt to stimulate and develop the muscles of pelvic floor.

Feed mount c=1 r=2

This is a small connector between the fresh gas outlet connector (FGO) on an anaesthetic machine and the tubing used to connect to the patient or ventilator. Both ends are normally push fit.

Fibre-optic light source n=10 c=3

Illumination within the cavities of the body during endoscopy is usually provided using a flexible fibre-optic light pipe within the endoscope coupled to a high-intensity light source outside the body. The light source is a standard piece of operating theatre equipment with a receptacle to accommodate the fibre bundles from various types of endoscope. Inside the unit is one or more high-intensity tungsten filament lamps, usually fan cooled, and a lens system to focus the light on to the end of the fibre bundle. Some devices include a xenon tube to provide high-intensity flashes for photographic endoscopy.

These are sometimes called cold light sources since a high-intensity illumination can be provided without heat in the endoscope. Previously endoscopes used small bulbs which had to operate inside the body. These were very troublesome. Using a fibre-optic light source it is possible to

109

obtain very high levels of illumination with proper colour balance of the image. This is particularly important in some examinations (e.g. within the bladder).

Fibre-optic recorder n=2 c=5 r=3

A strip chart recorder of exceptionally high frequency response (up to 100 kHz) can be made by projecting the spot from a cathode ray tube on to a moving strip of photographic paper. An effective way of achieving this is with a special CRT in which the glass face plate is made up of short optic fibres so that the luminous spot on the inside of the glass transfers its light along the fibres to the outside where the glass is in contact with the photographic strip. In medical work such recorders are used for electromyography, where frequency response requirement is about 1 kHz.

They are also employed in echo-cardiography where the single line scan showing bright dots representing echoes received is presented to the fibre-optic CRT. The paper record will show not only the echoes received, but also their motion.

Fibrillator n=1 c=2 r=7

This is an instrument for arresting the action of the heart prior to cardiac surgery. The heart is usually put into ventricular fibrillation by a medium-frequency sine wave stimulation through electrodes on the surface of the heart.

Fick cardiac output computer r=9

One of the many important measurements undertaken during cardiac catheterization procedures is a calculation of the rate of blood flow from the heart (cardiac output) in litres/minute. This is often achieved by injecting an indicator material into the pulmonary artery from the tip of the cardiac catheter and detecting the concentration of this material as it passes through the peripheral arteries.

An alternative method which does not require an indicator to be introduced is the Fick method in which the indicator is oxygen. The rate of use of oxygen is determined by a spirometer in conjunction with a carbon dioxide absorber. The patient rebreathes the air from the spirometer and the total volume falls as oxygen is consumed, since the resulting carbon dioxide is absorbed in the soda-lime canister. At the same time, blood is sampled from the venous circulation (from the pulmonary artery) and from the arterial circulation (via a cannula in a peripheral artery) and the concentration of oxygen in the blood samples is determined using a cuvette oximeter.

Flow rate is then calculated as follows:

$$F = dm/dt \, /C_a - C_v$$

where F is the blood flow in litres/minute, dm/dt is the consumption of oxygen in litres/minute, C_a is the arterial concentration of oxygen in litres/litre and C_v is the venous concentration of oxygen in litres/litre.

The oxygen consumption may also be calculated using a fibre-optic oximeter which can be passed directly into the vessels.

Film badge n=200 c=1 r=3

It is required that all personnel who work with ionizing radiations wear monitors to log their accumulated exposure to radiation. The most common form of monitoring is the film badge in which a piece of photographic negative is covered by a set of filters which shade the film from incident radiation. At regular intervals the badges are returned to the monitoring service for development of the films and reading of the radiation dose from the optical density (opacity) of the film. The effect of the filters on the developed films is to allow an assessment of the type of radiation involved. This may be separated into diagnostic X-rays, radiotherapy, neutrons, and beta rays. The films are often read on automated densitometers but must also be examined visually, since radioisotope contamination may expose small spots on the film which might be missed by the densitometer.

For each film badge wearer, it is usual to maintain a cumulative total of radiation exposure which can be compared with accepted limits for daily or annual exposure.

Thermoluminescent dosimetry (TLD) badge systems provide an alternative.

Film changer n=3 c=4,5 r=7

Some X-ray procedures, such as cardiac or vascular investigations, require X-rays to be taken in rapid succession. In order to do this, a device is required to change the X-ray cassettes, or to move a large roll (e.g. 30 cm wide) of film, at sufficient speed. The difficulty of rapid film changing is compounded if bi-plane imaging is required and if simultaneous fluoroscopic screening is necessary.

Such devices are found in the X-ray department, particularly where cardiological investigations and angiography are undertaken. Such systems are not often found in use now.

Fistula monitor

During haemodialysis blood is normally drawn from, and returned to, a surgically created chamber (fistula) between an artery and a vein. A fistula monitor is normally used to monitor arterial blood pressure, and to prevent a blood pump from drawing more blood from a fistula than it is capable of providing. The monitor sometimes incorporates an air detection device to stop the blood pump should air be detected in the venous return blood tubing. On older machines a fistula monitor is often a separate device. Most modern machines include the device in the main console.

Flame photometer n=3 c=4 r=5,6,9

These are used in the clinical chemistry department to determine the concentration of pure metals, particularly sodium and potassium, in plasma and urine. They can be used in the emission or absorption mode by which they emit or absorb light at characteristic wavelengths for the atoms involved.

The emission flame photometer injects droplets of a diluted solution of a body fluid into a flame of propane or natural gas and air, under which conditions some metal elements emit light at characteristic wavelengths. The characteristic wavelengths for sodium are detected by a photometer after passing through a monochromator (prism or diffraction grating), or set of filters. Since the power of the light will depend on the rate of solution uptake, quality of aerosol production, and flame characteristics, calibration may be made against a lithium salt. Lithium does not normally occur in the human body and so the sodium and potassium spectral intensity may be compared with that detected for the known concentration of lithium.

Atomic absorption flame photometers work by passing a light of known spectral content through a flame in which the test sample is being ionized. The light source is usually a hollow cathode lamp coated with the metal which is to be determined. Thus the light passing through the beam contains the necessary spectral lines. It is important to differentiate between radiation generated in the flame and that absorbed by it and to achieve this the light source is pulsed so that the change in detected light is proportional to that absorbed in the flame. This device is sometimes called an atomic absorption spectrometer.

Flatbed recorder n=10 c=3,4 r=3

A pen recorder using broad paper usually with a potentiometric recording mechanism is used for recording slow variables (typically up to 1 Hz) such as those generated by analytical equipment in the pathology laboratory. Multichannel versions are available but they usually have a small error between the channels since the pens must not interfere with each other as they cross over.

112

Fleisch tube n=3 c=2 r=6,9

This is the transducer used in a pneumotachograph for monitoring the flow of air in and out of the mouth. It consists of a wide bore tube in which there is a mesh or screen which slightly restricts the airflow through it. At each side of the mesh or screen there is a small tube, of two or three millimetres diameter, inserted into the airway, which is connected to a differential pressure transducer. The resistance to flow presented by the screen produces a differential pressure which is proportional to the airflow through the device.

Theoretical problems exist because the inspired and expired volumes and gas mixtures are not the same, so that the pressure drop will not be the same for equal flow in each direction. Also, water vapour in the expired gases may condense on the mesh unless heating is applied, or some other anti-condensation measure is used.

Fleisch tubes are used in equipment for lung function testing and also in connection with artificial lung ventilation systems.

Flexoplate r=2

Traditionally monopolar surgical diathermy has been conducted using an indifferent electrode made of lead and wrapped in a saline-soaked gauze. Satisfactory results can be obtained using a Flexoplate, which is a dry electrode, provided intimate contact with the skin can be maintained. Since dry skin is a good electrical insulator, the Flexoplate (this is in fact a trade name) works by capacitance, which presents only a small impedance to the electric current at the frequencies used for surgical diathermy. It is usually made of plastic-backed metal foil, is about 10 cm square, and the foil is cut in a special pattern to permit the use of a Flexoplate monitor in the diathermy set to recognize accidental disconnection of the indifferent electrode connections.

The plate is normally applied around the thigh by a wide bandage or an inflatable cuff.

Flexoplate monitor n=10 c=1 r=2

A number of injuries to patients have been caused by the loss of connection to the indifferent electrode during the use of monopolar surgical diathermy. One way of reducing this possibility with the flexible type of dry indifferent electrode (Flexoplate), is to have two connectors and two wires to the machine. Inside the diathermy set the Flexoplate monitor passes a small current up one wire, through the foil of the electrode and back to the machine. If this current is interrupted due to a disconnection then an alarm sounds and the apparatus may be temporarily disabled. Modern surgical diathermy machines have this facility built in.

Floating electrode r=3,9

Even the best electrodes for picking up potentials from the skin for ECG, EEG and EMG cause artefacts when there is movement. The movement changes the quality of contact between the electrode and skin, thus affecting the electrode potential and resistance.

This problem can be reduced by mounting the electrode a short distance from the skin on a plastic washer, and filling the recess with electrode jelly. This is called a floating electrode, or a fluid column electrode.

Flow-directed catheter r=4

Catheters for measuring pressure for cardiac output can be positioned deep within the arterial system by allowing the movement of blood to assist a small balloon, mounted on the catheter, to lead it to the required position within the heart or major vessels. The Swan-Ganz catheter is an example of a flow-directed catheter which can be passed from a peripheral artery through the chambers of the heart and into the pulmonary artery. From here it can be moved to wedge in a smaller vessel in the pulmonary vascular system for measuring pressure in the capillary bed (wedge pressure). Other catheters may be used for measuring pressures, or for delivering or sampling dye in the great vessels or in the coronary artery, for cardiac output measurement or X-ray contrast procedures.

A major advantage of flow-directed catheters is that they can be positioned without using fluoroscopy and may thus be used in intensive care as well as in the cardiac catheter laboratory. They can also be left in position in order to monitor changes in pressure or cardiac output.

Flowmeter n=500 c=1 r=2

This may refer to blood flowmeters such as ultrasonic and electromagnetic types but usually the term is reserved for gas flowmeters as used in anaesthetic apparatus. There are various types such as the Wright's respirometer but the most common type is the rotameter used on anaesthetic machines which have a rotating bobbin in a tapered glass tube. The gas flow rate is indicated by the height in the glass tube at which the bobbin rotates. A cheaper form is the ball float meter.

Fluorescence spectrometer n=1 c=4,5 r=9

This is similar to a fluorimeter (fluorometer) but employs a diffraction grating in place of a filter. This enables the identity and concentration of fluorescent materials within a test sample to be determined from the spectral lines present in the emitted light.

Such devices are used in the clinical chemistry laboratory for estimation of the concentration of some of the chemicals which occur in body fluids. A few of these are fluorescent and their concentrations can be determined by measuring the quantity of light emitted at their characteristic frequencies when illuminated by another (usually shorter) wavelength. Some materials are naturally fluorescent but other chemicals may be identified by combining with a fluorescent reagent. See Fluorimeter.

Fluorimeter (fluorometer) n=3 c=5 r=5,9

The fluorimeter or fluorometer is an instrument used in the clinical chemistry laboratory to determine the concentration of particular substances in samples of body fluids. The instrument is based on the property of some molecules to emit light in a characteristic spectrum when illuminated by light of another (usually shorter) wavelength. The fluorescent materials may be in the samples to be analysed or they may be produced by combination with reagents.

The normal layout for the instrument is a slit-lamp light source (often ultraviolet), a filter to make sure that the expected fluorescent spectrum is not present in the illuminating light, and a cuvette containing the sample. Very dilute samples are used since this avoids re-absorption of the light produced and is also economical in the required quantity of the sample. The light emitted is normally detected at right angles from the incident light through a secondary filter to the photometer.

Not many materials exhibit fluorescence, but those that do can be determined by fluorometry, with much greater sensitivity than by using a spectrophotometer. The principal disadvantage of fluorometry is the sensitivity of its determinations to temperature and pH of the sample.

Fluoroscope

Direct viewing of X-ray images, including moving images, has been achieved using a fluorescent screen placed in front of the patient. The X-rays cause the screen to glow in response to the X-ray intensity so that the image can be seen in very low light. Later developments on this idea have been to transfer the image on to cine film, on to a television picture or video recorder. In these cases the screen and translation mechanism is known as an image intensifier, which is an electronic device for increasing the brightness of the image to a level suitable for photography or video. Fluoroscopy now refers to the whole process of presenting a moving X-ray picture on a television screen or on to cine film. The term 'screening unit' is often applied to X-ray apparatus with fluoroscopic capability. These may be mobile units, or major static units.

Although fluoroscopy is extremely useful for many procedures, the sharpness of the image is poor compared with direct imaging on film.

Fluotec n=40 c=2 r=2

This is a trade name for a type of temperature-compensated vaporizer which fits into the back bar of an anaesthetic machine to deliver a controlled concentration of halothane into the carrier gas (usually nitrous oxide and oxygen). The Mk2, now being phased out, has poor accuracy at low gas flow rates. The Mk3 and Mk4 versions improve on this.

FM tape recorder n=2 c=4 r=3

Ordinary direct recording (DR) tape recorders cannot record continuous or slow-moving signals and are therefore unsuitable for recording most biological signals. This problem can be overcome by using a carrier signal. In an FM (frequency modulated) recorder this is a tone which has a frequency which can be recorded on a direct recording machine (e.g. 1 kHz), and the signal to be recorded causes the frequency of the tone to change. For instance an input signal of 1 V may cause the tone to move to 2 kHz and a 2 V signal may move it to 3 kHz. When the recording is played back, a frequency to voltage converter will decode the signal, back into the original voltages, for off-line analysis or for demonstration purposes. Clearly the played back frequencies must be a faithful reproduction of those presented during recording and this requires a very stable tape speed, or a compensating mechanism, so that variations in tape speed are identified and a correction factor applied to the output signals.

Biological variables such as pressures, ECG, EEG, blood flow, blood gas tension, etc. may be recorded on an FM tape recorder and replayed for analysis. FM tape recorders are less used than a few years ago because of the capability of some modern computing equipment to perform high speed analysis of signals in real time. They would be found in the physics and bioengineering departments, in some clinical research units and possibly in the intensive care department.

Foetal electrocardiograph r=9

The ECG signal from the foetal heart can be detected on the abdomen of the mother, or directly from an electrode on the scalp of the foetus, as soon as this is exposed through the cervix during the first stage of labour. The heart rate information so derived is used during labour to monitor the state of the foetus, since the fluctuations in rate which occur as a result of uterine contractions provide an important indicator of foetal wellbeing. Scalp electrodes are used and these may be small suction cups with a spike electrode at the centre, small metal 'crocodile' jaws squeezed together with a special tool on to the foetal scalp, or a sharp wire screw which is rotated to pass into the skin of the scalp.

If the ECG is detected through the abdominal wall of the mother then the signal is very small and is subject to interference from the ECG of the mother. Electronic processing may enable a separation of the two so that foetal heart rate can be monitored at earlier stages of pregnancy. It is more common now to use doppler ultrasound foetal heart detectors in both of these applications until the foetal scalp is well exposed during labour when the scalp electrode is the preferred method of monitoring the rate.

The foetal electrocardiograph is normally incorporated into an instrument which also monitors the uterine contractions, and the whole instrument is called a cardiotocograph or a foetal heart monitor.

Foetal heart detector n=10 c=2 r=1

This is usually an ultrasonic doppler device although early types were low-frequency microphones applied to the maternal abdomen. Ultrasonic types employ a low frequency of ultrasound (e.g 2 MHz) transmitted through the skin as a continuous wave (not pulsed); the echoes returning from the region of the foetal heart are shifted in frequency due to the movement of the walls and valves of the heart and also the blood. The doppler shifts from the transmitted ultrasonic frequency fall mostly in the low audible range and so, by a simple process of frequency subtraction, these doppler frequencies are presented to a loudspeaker. The foetal heart rate can be detected by timing the rate of pulsations, and some information about the placenta can also be gained by the characteristic sound produced by the blood flowing slowly through this organ. Foetal heart detectors of the above type have to some extent replaced the traditional foetal stethoscope and are found commonly in the labour rooms and the antenatal clinics.

Foetal monitor/recorder n=10 c=4,5

This is essentially a device for recording the uterine contractions during labour, and also the foetal heart rate on a beat-to-beat basis, to monitor the progress of labour, and in particular the wellbeing of the foetus. The instrument is sometimes called a cardiotocograph. Uterine contractions are usually monitored using a tocodynamometer lightly strapped on to the mother's abdomen and this consists of a central plunger coupled to a force transducer and outer guard ring so that the plunger is pressed during the uterine contractions. This provides a qualitative indication of the strength and occurrence of contractions and this is compared with the foetal heart rates which result. Sometimes an internal transducer is used once the foetal membranes have been ruptured and a recording catheter can be introduced into the uterus. The recording catheter can be a fluid-filled tube connected to an external pressure transducer or it may have a miniature pressure transducer built into the tip of the catheter.

Foetal heart rate is normally monitored by a foetal scalp electrode clamped or screwed into the foetal scalp when exposed through the opening cervix. Alternative methods of recording the foetal heart rate are to have electrodes on the mother's abdomen or by an ultrasonic transducer detecting the blood flow and other movements in the foetal heart.

The records are presented on a paper trace to identify both the effects of the contractions on foetal heart rate and the trend of these effects. In some modern instruments, computer processing is applied to these signals, to provide time compression to be applied for a display indicating the trend of these parameters during the course of labour.

Foetal monitors are used in the labour ward but variations on these machines are used in the antenatal clinic to assess the state of the foetus in other phases of pregnancy.

Fogging machine n=1 c=3 r=2

This is a large nebulizer designed to provide a mist of a sterilizing agent for the sterilization of a whole room. The technique is not particularly effective and is not often used.

Force plate/platform n=1 c=5

The assessment of walking, and the study of the functioning of artificial hips and knees, artificial legs, and external support mechanisms (orthoses), can be assisted by the use of a force plate. Also known as a walking platform, this device consists of a metal plate held by a strong suspension in a frame with strain gauges to measure the forces applied by the foot in three directions, and also the rotational forces.

The apparatus may come with the necessary strain gauge amplifiers, and with a computer and programs to resolve the forces and moments, and to provide graphical display of the results. Such a device might be used in the orthopaedic surgery or limb-fitting department.

Formalin sterilizing unit/cabinet n=3 c=4 r=2

Surgical instruments and some larger items of equipment can be sterilized in a special cabinet into which formalin vapour is introduced. This may be a passive system in which the formalin is poured into trays to evaporate slowly or it may be nebulized and blown on to the equipment. Large cabinet types exist into which a whole trolley can be wheeled, such as an anaesthetic machine, ventilator or baby incubator, and which are fitted with a flue to exhaust the excess vapour to the outside air.

The whole process takes several hours and some preparation is required beforehand. The method is not regarded as ideal since there is no guarantee of penetration of the whole equipment system. Examples of formalin sterilization cabinets are the Drager Aseptor and the Vickers formalin disinfection unit.

Frame-freeze module r=1

This is a device to retain a single still image from a moving sequence. Most video recorders can provide this facility though the results are not always satisfactory.

Real-time ultrasonic scanners usually include a frame-freeze facility although this is usually achieved with a digital scan converter in which each frame of the moving image is stored in a computer-type memory. The contents of the memory are being read on to the display screen at a high rate and the image can be frozen at any time by arresting the flow of new information to the memory. The facility is used during real-time scanning for examination or recording. Since the image is stored in a computer memory it is also possible to further operate on the image to improve or change the contrast ratio, to improve the sharpness of the image, or to make calculations of distance, circumference, or area to establish the size of the organs or areas of interest.

Fraser Sweatman pin safety system r=2

Vaporizers for volatile anaesthetic agents are normally temperature compensated and calibrated for a single agent. If the vaporizer is filled with the wrong agent the calibration will be incorrect, perhaps with lethal consequences. As an attempt to limit the possibility of the use of incorrect agents the Fraser Sweatman pin safety system provides connectors between the filling bottles and the vaporizers which cannot be interchanged. The filling bottles have a screw thread which can only be mated with the correct filling nozzle.

Free-field audiometer n=3 c=4

This is an audiometer which presents the test sounds to the patient through loudspeakers rather than through headphones. In at least one sense this is a more natural form of presentation but the test environment must be extremely quiet if it is required to identify small hearing losses. The test environment may also affect the results by creating standing waves and excessive reverberation. Therefore some free field audiometers produce a fluctuating frequency (see Warble tone audiometer) which minimizes these effects. Speech audiometry may also be performed in the free field.

Frenzel glasses n=1 c=1

One of the standard tests in the investigation of dizziness or vertigo involves asking the patient to look in different directions while the clinician observes the patient's eyes in order to detect an abnormal eye movement called nystagmus. In the normal clinical environment, only patients with acute vestibular problems will exhibit this particular symptom since their eyes will be held steady by observation of the surroundings. A much more sensitive test is to do this in darkness and there are several methods by which the patient's eye movement can be detected. The best method of achieving this is to use an electronystagmograph, although an infrared viewer, or Frenzel glasses, will also allow a subjective assessment of eye movement.

Frenzel glasses comprise a pair of very thick lenses which serve to completely blur the patient's observed environment while giving the clinician a magnified view of the patient's eyes. Two small bulbs built into the frames illuminate the patient's eyes. The advantages of Frenzel glasses over the electronystagmograph and infrared viewer, are low cost and that a totally dark environment is not required, although subdued lighting in the room enhances the effect.

Fuel cell oxygen analyser n=10 c=2,3 r=6

These are used for measuring oxygen concentration in anaesthetic and therapeutic gases, and can also be adapted for blood oxygen measurement. As the name implies, this is essentially a small electrical generating cell which requires oxygen to enable the chemical reaction to take place. It uses potassium hydroxide as the electrolyte contained behind an oxygen permeable membrane (usually PTFE – Teflon) with a gold-plated sintered steel cathode and a lead anode.

They are relatively slow acting and the cell has a limited life depending on oxygen exposure. They can be made to fit into a T-piece in an anaesthetic circuit.

Fumigation unit r=2

Some equipment and surgical instruments may be disinfected or sterilized in a fumigation unit, usually employing formalin in a special cabinet. This may be a rack for the instruments held in perforated trays over flat trays containing formalin, or it may be a closed cabinet into which a whole trolley can be wheeled carrying an anaesthetic machine, ventilator, infant incubator or even an operating table. In these larger types the formalin may be nebulized and blown into the apparatus inside, and they may have a flue to remove the vapour from the room. The technique is not ideal but may provide the only practical solution for large systems. Examples of the larger systems are the Drager Aseptor, and the Vickers formalin disinfection unit.

Functional electrical stimulator (FES) n=5 c=2 r=4

Lost nerve or muscle function can be supplemented or replaced by a neural prosthesis. Functional electrical stimulation (FES) may be used for foot drop correction, stimulation of the legs for gait improvement in cerebral palsy, correction of curvature of the spine, diaphragm pacing for the stimulation of breathing via the phrenic nerve, or the restoration of the micturition reflex.

Most of these techniques are in the early stages of development and may be simple asynchronous devices, or may use pressure, force, or EMG input to regulate their action.

The devices themselves are simple electrical pulse stimulators employing a variety of pulse rates, pulse lengths, and operating currents and may be applied externally or internally via transcutaneous connections or via inductive loops.

Functional residual capacity (FRC) analyser n=2 c=4,5 r=9

This device may be part of a general lung function analysis system or it may be an independent instrument. There are three techniques in use to establish the residual capacity of the lungs as follows:

1. By nitrogen washout in which the patient is connected to a spirometer at the end of expiration, and draws in a gas mixture containing no nitrogen (pure oxygen is often used). The patient makes several breaths in and out of the spirometer, exhaling oxygen, carbon dioxide, nitrogen and water vapour. The eventual proportion of nitrogen in the breathed gases can be used to estimate the original end-expiratory volume of the lungs and airways (FRC). Nitrogen is measured by sampling off-line.
2. A quantity of a tracer gas which is not absorbed in the lungs (e.g. helium) may be introduced into the inspired air and the concentration achieved in the expired air measured. This will allow an estimation of functional residual capacity. The patient may breath into a spirometer to allow

proper mixing of the helium, in which case the volume of the spirometer must be taken into account in the calculation. The helium concentration may be determined by using radioactive helium (see Helium FRC analyser), or by use of a katharometer.

3. Alternatively a total body plethysmograph (TBP) may be used in which the patient is enclosed in a chamber (body box) so that changes in the volume, flow or pressure of the breathed gases, and changes in volume of the whole body may be estimated.

G

Galvanometric recorder n=50 c=3,4,5 r=3

This is a type of chart recorder using pens which are deflected by a moving coil mechanism (galvanometer) similar to those employed in most electrical meters. A small coil of wire is mounted on a spindle between the poles of a powerful magnet. When an electric current passes through the wires of the coil it forces the spindle to rotate. If this rotation is restrained by a spring the angle through which it turns is proportional to the current through the coil. In galvanometric recorders the input signal is amplified and delivered as a current to the coil of the galvanometer. A pointer attached to the end of the spindle marks the recording paper to indicate the magnitude of the input signal. The marks may be made by ink (the pointer is a narrow tube through which ink is forced), or it may write by pressure or heat on special paper. Some types do not have a pointer but spray the ink from a hole in the spindle or have a small mirror mounted on the spindle or coil which reflects light on to a photographic paper. These latter types can operate at higher frequencies (e.g. 1 kHz) because of their very low inertial mass.

Galvanometric pen recorders are widely used for recording ECG, EEG, blood pressure and other signals with frequency components up to 100 Hz, and are thus found in many hospital departments as single or multichannel instruments. The mirror and ink jet recorders may be used for electromyography (EMG) or other applications where the wider bandwidth is important.

A small defect with the pen types is that the pen draws an arc on the paper and not a straight line. Straight line recording is usually achieved by feeding the paper over a 'knife edge' writing bar, but this introduces a linearity error at the extremes of deflection. There would be approximately 10% error at 30 degrees deflection.

Gamma camera n=3 c=8 r=3

This is used in the nuclear medicine or X-ray department for producing a picture of the distribution of radiopharmaceuticals in the body or in particular organs. Individual images can be acquired rapidly into a computer memory, and so it is possible to build up a set of images to show the passage of a particular radiopharmaceutical. The gamma camera is a major advance

123

on the rectilinear scanner since it does not require the head to move to produce a two-dimensional image.

The principal components of a gamma camera are a large sodium iodide crystal coupled to a parallel hole collimator, and a set of photomultiplier (PM) tubes mounted above the crystal. Gamma rays pass through the holes in the collimator and cause flashes of light in the crystal at locations corresponding to their points of origin in the body. The location of the scintillations is calculated by computer from the strengths of light received by the various PM tubes.

Ganzfeld stimulator n=1 c=4,5

In order to measure the electrical responses of the eye and visual system an optical (flash) stimulator is required. The Ganzfeld stimulator is designed to provide a uniform light stimulus to the whole of the visual field for use in electroretinography (ERG) and visual evoked cortical response (VER or VEP). Although the most commonly used stimulus is a high-intensity, short-duration flash of white light, control of the flash brightness and colour is available, as is the level of steady background illumination.

The Ganzfeld stimulator comprises a hemisphere, typically 50 cm in diameter, into which the patient looks. The eyes are held at the approximate centre of the hemisphere by placing the chin on a rest. The inside of the hemisphere is made of white translucent material and the flash is provided by a strobe and set of colour filters mounted behind this. The strobe timing, intensity and selection of colour filters are often controlled electronically. A small central fixation light is provided in the rear wall, and additional red lights may be included at each side of this to allow electro-oculography (EOG) to be performed. In this test the two side fixation lights are illuminated alternately and the patient is asked to look at whichever light is on.

Such devices are found in the ophthalmology department or in the neurophysiology department.

Gas cylinder n=500 c=1 r=2

Medical gases for therapy or anaesthesia are supplied by pipeline or in bottles (cylinders). The cylinders are steel, very heavy and strong enough to contain the enormous pressures required to get enough gas into a small volume. At the pressures used, some gases liquefy, and therefore behave differently during storage and delivery. Oxygen (1980 psi) and Entonox (1980 psi) remain gases, while nitrous oxide (639 psi), carbon dioxide (723 psi), and cyclopropane (64 psi) liquefy. The liquids will cool considerably during expansion and this may cause problems, although this drawback is put to good use in cryosurgery where nitrous oxide evaporation and expansion is used as the energy source. In the case of Entonox, it should not be stored below freezing point (0°C) since the mixture (50/50 nitrous oxide and oxygen) may separate.

Medical gas cylinders, when empty, are exchanged for full ones by a commercial medical gas company. The fullness of the cylinder is determined by the pressure (in the case of gases), or by weight (in the case of the liquefied gases).

The top of the cylinder has a tapered thread into which is fitted a valve, usually turned by a special key. The gas outlet from this valve is connected to a pressure reducing valve and pressure gauge and other devices depending on the application. Cylinders for use with anaesthetic apparatus usually have a pin-index system on the valve block to ensure that only the correct gas can be connected to each port (yoke) on the machine. Medical gas cylinders are also colour coded but unfortunately there is no international agreement as yet.

The UK standards for cylinder coding are set out in BS 1319 (1976). The common codes are listed in Table 3.

Table 3 Colour codes for medical gas cylinders

Gas	Colour – valve end	Cylinder body
Oxygen	White	Black
Nitrous oxide	Blue	Blue
Cyclopropane	Orange	Orange
Carbon dioxide	Grey	Grey
Nitrogen	Black	Grey
Medical air	White and black	Grey
Entonox	White and blue	Blue

Gas-liquid chromatograph (GLC) n=3 c=4 r=9

A sample of body fluid, usually blood, is purified to some extent and then added to an organic solvent before being flash vaporized and fed into a column of solid material (e.g. diatomaceous earth) which may be a few millimetres in diameter and 1 metre long. A carrier gas (usually nitrogen or helium) is also injected into the column which sweeps the evaporated sample down the column. A detector at the end of the column provides an electrical output proportional to the quantity of the compound found in the effluent gas. A number of types of detector are available which include ionization detectors, thermal conductivity detectors, and electron capture detectors. Ionization detectors are most commonly used in clinical laboratory applications. The electrical output is fed to a recorder which shows a number of peaks of output corresponding to particular materials, commonly drugs.

Gas–liquid chromatographs can work with very small samples with great sensitivity and produce complete analyses of important substances in less than one hour.

Gas mixing valve r=4

This is a device to mix oxygen and air, or nitrous oxide and oxygen, before delivery. This may be a gas adder, an entrainment device, or blender. Many such devices may be used in anaesthetic or oxygen therapy apparatus which have different properties of interaction between the delivered flow rate and the relative pressure sources of the two gases. They normally employ pressure regulators, and separate or dual needle valves to change the proportions of each gas.

Gastric pump n=1 c=3,4

Stomach washout may be achieved by the simple procedure of passing a tube into the stomach and pouring in fluid through a funnel, and then lowering the tube to siphon out the contents. Automated versions exist which provide a washing cycle, and such devices may also be adapted for investigation purposes in which samples of stomach contents are removed at intervals into vials for examination. Such devices would contain a small suction pump, timer, and the necessary tubes, filters, and jars.

Gastroscope n=5 c=4 r=4

The examination or treatment of sites within the stomach, oesophagus and small intestines may be achieved using a long flexible endoscope employing fibre-optic transmission of illuminating light and the image from within the gut to an eyepiece at the distal end. Controls at the telescope end enable the tip to be manipulated to the position required.

The endoscope contains extra channels for the infusion or withdrawal of liquid or gas, or for the passage of sampling catheters or instruments for electrosurgery, laser surgery, and for cutting, grasping, and crushing. The introduction of flexible endoscopes has enabled many surgical treatments to be undertaken without entry through the skin. For instance, the treatment of ulcers and in particular the control of bleeding can be achieved by a relatively minor operation from the point of view of the patient.

Geiger–Müller tube r=3

This is a particularly sensitive form of ionization chamber filled with neon or argon gas at a low pressure. The electrodes are a central wire, surrounded by a metal tube, between which a high voltage is applied. A detectable electric current may flow following ionization of a single particle of gas since the acceleration of the ions towards the electrodes causes further ionization. These tubes may be used in radiation detectors, particularly for detecting and estimating the activity of radio nuclides.

Glottograph n=1 c=2,3

A glottograph is another name for a laryngograph which displays an analogue of the movement of the vocal cords, derived from the impedance between two electrodes on the skin over the glottis. These are used in the speech therapy department to assist patients to make sounds correctly with the larynx. An alternative instrument exists (photoelectric glottograph) which registers the area of opening between the vocal cords in the vertical plane.

Goldman inhaler c=1 r=2

An anaesthetic nosepiece for dental anaesthesia. It has a removable edge pad which can be replaced when perished or damaged. The Oxford inhaler is a similar device.

Goldman vaporizer c=2 r=2

A low resistance type of halothane or trichloroethylene vaporizer for use in dental anaesthesia in a demand flow analgesia circuit.

Goniometer n=5 c=2,3

This is a general term for a device measuring angles. In medical work they are encountered in orthopaedics for measuring the flexion of joints and tilt of the spine. They may be simple mechanical devices of the pendulum type, some of which may be designed to show on X-ray images, or electronic types including optical polarizing filters or light reflectors.

Grentz-ray set n=1 c=6

This is a therapy X-ray set which emits low-energy X-rays in the range of 10–100 kV. These sets will usually be used with open-ended applicators which are brought into contact with the skin, thus defining focal point to skin distance (FSD). The higher energies are used for treating superficial skin lesions and the lower energies for treating very superficial lesions and some skin disorders. Grentz-ray sets will be found in radiotherapy centres and in some skin clinics.

Grey scale display unit $r=1$

A type of display or paper recorder utilizing varying intensity to indicate a third parameter. This is best known in medical equipment in grey scale display of ultrasonic images in which the brightness is used to indicate the intensity of the echo. Grey scale displays on CRTs can be achieved using a conventional CRT for real-time scanning or using scan converters with TV-type displays. Fibre-optic recorders can also achieve grey scale printing of such images on photographic paper.

Grommet

Also known as a dottle or stopple, this is a small plastic (PTFE) tube which is inserted in a hole made in the eardrum by an ENT surgeon. It serves to keep the hole open for ventilation and draining purposes following surgical drainage of the middle ear.

Guard ring tocograph $n=8$ $c=1$ $r=9$

Usually a crude form of applanation tonometer used for monitoring the contractions of the uterus during labour. It consists of a ring about 5 cm in diameter surrounding a springloaded plunger connected to a force or displacement transducer. The whole device is held on to the abdomen with an elastic strap so that pressure variations in the uterus are transmitted to the plunger. These devices are usually met as the 'contractions transducer' with a foetal cardiotocograph.

Although these devices are sometimes used to provide quantitative information about uterine contractions they are very much prone to error or operational difficulties which make them more suited to non-quantitative applications. The alternative is the use of internal uterine pressure measurement via a fluid-filled catheter, balloon catheter or micro-transducer. However, each of these has its own problems. Use of quantitative information about uterine contractions to control the delivery of labour-inducing drugs has been restricted, partly due to these shortcomings.

Gustometer $n=1$ $c=1,2$

Also known as a taste tester or electrogustometer, this device is a direct current electrical stimulator for measuring the threshold of taste by passing a small d.c. current from one side of the tongue to either the tip of the tongue or another midline point on the cranium (e.g. the nose). The threshold current should be approximately equal on each side of the tongue. A significant inequality may be suggestive of a lesion affecting the fifth cranial (trigeminal) nerve. Gustometers are sometimes used in the neurophysiology or ENT departments for differential diagnosis of Bell's palsy.

H

Haematocrit centrifuge n=7 c=3,4 r=3

The haematocrit is the volume percentage of the red blood cells in blood and is determined in the haematology department. The centrifuge is usually small and may hold up to 50 samples in tiny pipettes mounted radially on a high-speed rotating disc. The cells and the plasma, having different density, are separated by the centrifuging process. The haematocrit is determined after centrifuging by measuring the relative lengths of the red (cell) and yellow (plasma) sections of the tubes.

Haemacytometer/haemocytometer n=3 c=5

Haemacytometer, or haemocytometer is another name for a blood cell counter. The term may be used to describe traditional apparatus using a microscope and manual counting, often with a special slide with a graticule, or applied to automatic counters such as the Coulter or Fisher devices.

Haemodialysis machine n=20 c=5 r=3,4

This is commonly called an 'artificial kidney'. It is a system of pumps, clamps, timers, tubing circuitry, and heaters, which passes blood from the patient, and a dialysate solution, through a dialyser. Usually the system manufactures the dialysate by mixing a concentrated solution with filtered, softened or de-ionized tap water. This is heated to blood temperature, de-aerated and checked for conductivity before passing through the dialyser where it flows over a semipermeable membrane. The patient's blood is made to pass over the other side of the membrane so that fluids and toxins of low molecular weight can pass from the blood into the dialysate. Other molecules from the dialysate pass into the blood to rectify imbalances before it passes to waste. Blood is drawn from, and returned to the patient at a shunt or fistula between blood vessels of an arm, leg, or other access point.

Haemodialysis machines are used in hospitals in cases of acute renal failure and also in some cases of poisoning (e.g. drug overdoses). Patients with chronic renal failure are usually treated using machines at their homes or at special dialysis centres.

Since the patient's life depends upon the correct functioning of the machine it contains a number of measuring and alarm circuits including a conductivity meter which identifies the correct concentration of the dialysing fluid, a temperature monitor to ensure that the dialysate neither cools nor heats the blood, and a dialysate pressure monitor since the quantity of water withdrawn from the patient will depend upon the pressure differential between the blood and dialysate.

Because of the pressure differential, or incorrect assembly of the dialyser, the membrane may rupture leading to a blood leak into the dialysate. A blood leak detector, which is essentially an optical densitometer, is always included in the dialysate circuit after the artificial kidney.

In the circuit containing the patient's blood, the pressure of the blood returning to the patient (venous pressure) is measured, to give protection against leaks in the blood lines, and a special monitor is required to ensure that no air is passed to the patient. This may be a blood level detector on the bubble trap, or another optical densitometer or ultrasonic bubble detector to identify the presence of bubbles in the return circuit to the patient.

Haemofiltration apparatus n=1 c=5 r=4

As a variation of haemodialysis for treatment of acute kidney failure a different kind of dialysing membrane can be used to provide the transfer of large quantities of fluid (15–80 litres) from the body by ultrafiltration. At the same time transfer of small and medium-sized molecules takes place with much higher clearance rates of larger molecules than occurs with haemo-dialysis. The fluid loss is made up before or after the haemofiltration using a specially prepared electrolyte (Ringer's solution).

The technique is expensive to use, but appropriate in some disorders.

Haemoheater n=20 c=2

This is another name for a blood warmer used to elevate the temperature of blood to body heat during transfusion. They are usually heated water baths through which the blood is passed in a coiled tube although dry types exist in which the blood passes through a coil or bag enclosed between two heated plates. Electronic circuits control the temperature and provide protection against overheating.

Haemoperfusion apparatus r=4

Removal of toxins from the blood, particularly in renal failure, may be achieved by passing the blood over material which absorbs (or adsorbs) a specific toxin or specific range of toxins. The material is usually activated carbon coated with cellulose, to reduce damage to the blood. As yet, such devices are not sufficiently well developed for normal clinical use except for the treatment of poisoning.

Haemotonometer n=5 c=3 r=6

Literally this just means a blood pressure meter but the term has been coined to refer to a double cuff indirect blood pressure meter which works on a principle somewhat similar to an oscillotonometer. Pulsations in pressure in each cuff are detected by thermistors in the connecting tubes. There are no pulsations in either cuff when inflated above the systolic pressure. There is a time (phase) difference in the pulsations in each cuff at pressures between systolic and diastolic pressures and no phase difference at pressures below diastolic. These various possibilities can be decoded electronically.

Such devices may exist as independent instruments or be incorporated into general monitors, sometimes called vital signs monitors which are used during anaesthesia to provide a number of measurements (including blood pressure) simultaneously.

Haldane apparatus c=2 r=2

An instrument for estimating the proportion of carbon dioxide in expired gases. A small sample of the gases is drawn into a calibrated burette and is then exposed to a solution of potassium hydroxide. The reduction of gas volume indicates the quantity of carbon dioxide absorbed by the potassium hydroxide. Such apparatus is used for calibration of electronic carbon dioxide monitors.

Hardening filter r=7

For a particular kV setting on an X-ray set the rays have a range of wavelengths, of which the shorter are less absorbed in tissue than the longer. The intensity of the longer wavelength rays can be reduced by the inclusion of a hardening filter in the X-ray beam. This is simply a sheet of aluminium or copper which attenuates the longer waves (soft rays) more than the shorter waves (hard rays), so that the beam reaching the patient has a higher proportion of hard rays.

It is the harder rays which pass through the patient and form the image, whereas the softer rays are absorbed in the patient, and can therefore be removed with advantage. The filters are sometimes shaped to absorb more of the energy near the centre of the beam in order to even out the intensity at the patient.

Head harness r=2

This can be an arrangement of elastic straps to hold a face mask on a patient during anaesthesia or intensive care. A similar arrangement may be used to hold the catheter and catheter mount when an endotracheal tube is in use. The term head-harness is also used sometimes to describe the frame used to hold the electrodes applied to the head for EEG recording.

Headphone

Usually used in pairs, with a headband, they have many applications, but have particular importance in audiology since most hearing tests are performed using an audiometer having both air conduction (using headphones) and bone conduction. Audiometric headphones are almost always electromagnetic (moving coil) devices and may be equipped with special noise-excluding ear muff surrounds for use when the ambient noise is too great to achieve accurate results. A common type in audiometric application is the Telephonics TDH39 (or 49) with MX41-AR cushions.

Hearing aid n=1000 c=1 r=3,4

A device for amplifying and delivering sound to the ear, (usually the better hearing of the two ears). Before 1930 these were passive devices, being variations of the 'hearing trumpet'. Since then they have developed with the various generations of electronics. Modern hearing aids are either body-worn microphones and amplifiers with a lead to an earpiece (strangely the earpiece is called a receiver), ear-level aids which fit behind the ear, housing both microphone and receiver, or even smaller devices which fit within the ear canal.

The frequency response of hearing aids is not flat. Sounds below 500 Hz are sharply attenuated and the output is also deficient in frequencies above 5 kHz (which are not required for speech intelligibility). Gain is usually nonlinear with increasing output and the typical full-on gain may be 60 dB. The microphone is usually an Electret type and the 'receiver' is usually a fixed coil and moving magnet type. If there is a defect in the mechanism which transmits sound from the ear drum to the cochlea (conductive deafness) sound is sometimes applied as vibrations through the mastoid bone just behind the ear. In this case the patient wears a head band or clip which causes the transducer to press on to the skin above the mastoid bone.

If one wears a hearing aid for a few minutes, the shortcomings become obvious. They are monaural (although sometimes two are worn) and there may be considerable distortion, resulting in harsh sound, but more serious is the intermodulation distortion. This means that when more than one sound is present (e.g. a motor car and a voice) the result is a jumble of sound which may be very difficult to make sense of. The amplifier is unlikely to have the required dynamic range to handle low and high sound levels at the same time or in rapid succession. Thus, clipping may be employed to limit the peak amplitude, or in more complex devices there may be an automatic gain circuit. This results in less distortion of larger signals but may have other undesirable effects, such as total loss of output following a large impulse of sound.

An aid with the required performance characteristics for each patient is chosen following clinical assessment and an audiogram. The effectiveness in use depends to a large extent on the quality of fitting of the ear mould.

Hearing aid test box n=1 c=4,5

Audiology departments need to test the performance of hearing aids to ensure their correct operation and assess the effect of their preset controls. The hearing aid test box comprises a small acoustically treated chamber (which may be bench-top size or free standing), an audio oscillator, amplifier, loudspeaker (within the chamber), 2 cc coupler, microphone and sound level metering circuitry. The hearing aid is placed within the calibrated sound field within the chamber, and its output is monitored with the 2 cc coupler, microphone and metering system. Measurements can be taken at several discrete frequencies or by sweeping the test frequency continuously throughout the required range (typically 250 Hz to 5 kHz). The usual tests include measurement of the gain of the hearing aid, maximum output and frequency response, although distortion measurements are sometimes included.

Heart-assist device r=4

This may be an intra-aortic balloon or a blood pump. Intra-aortic balloons are positioned in the descending aorta via an incision in the femoral artery and assist the heart by inflating during diastole and deflating during systole, triggered by the ECG. Blood pumps for assisting left ventricular action are usually based on the 'pusher plate' principle and may be pneumatic, hydraulic, or cam-driven. Since there is no space in the thorax for the device it can be implanted in the abdomen or can be external to the body. Operation can be triggered by the ECG.

Except for intra-aortic balloons, these devices are not in common use. The most common application is for patients unable to be weaned from pump-oxygenators.

Heart-lung machine n=2 c=5,6 r=4

This is a machine to replace the function of the heart and lungs during cardiac surgery, and is properly called a cardiopulmonary bypass machine. More details may be found under that heading.

Heart rate meter r=2

Heart rate meters display heart rate in beats/minute from the ECG signal, heart sounds, doppler ultrasound signal (such as in the foetal heart monitor), the peripheral (e.g. finger) pulse, or photo-plethysmograph signal.

It is often included (sometimes as an option) on cardioscopes, and the rate may be displayed on a meter, as a bar graph, or in figures on the monitor screen, or it may be presented as a graph of heart rate on a chart recorder.

Heart simulator r=4

This is often called a pulse duplicator and is a machine for testing artificial heart valves intended for implantation in the aortic and/or mitral position. It generates a pulsatile flow of a mixture (usually water–glycerol to provide equivalent viscosity, density, and Reynolds number to blood) through a model of the heart with the internal chambers created from a cast of a cadaver heart. Such devices may be used to visualize the flow patterns with different types of valve, often employing high-speed photography to track the movement of small particles suspended in the fluid. Pressures at various points in the system may be measured as well.

Pulse duplicators would be found in research laboratories to investigate the performance of valves during development or assessment of commercially available devices.

Heat camera n=1 c=6

There is a known relationship between the surface temperature of an object and its radiant power. This principle makes it possible to measure the temperature of a body without physical contact with it. Medical thermography is a technique whereby the temperature distribution on the surface of the body is mapped within a few tenths of a degree Kelvin. The human skin approximates to within 1% of a black body radiator and so a radiation thermometer can accurately detect the temperature of the skin. The detector in a radiation thermometer is typically arsenic trisulphide, indium antimonide, lead sulphide or thallium bromide iodine. The actual detector used will depend on the wavelengths (usually in the far infrared) required to be detected. Most thermography apparatus employs a mirror-type focusing device and the radiation beam is fed to the detector through a chopping disc which has a slot in it to interrupt the beam at a frequency of several hundred hertz so that an a.c. amplifier and phase sensitive detector can be used to amplify without the drift associated with d.c. amplifiers. See also Thermography apparatus.

The best known use of the heat camera or thermograph is in breast scanning, where irregularities in the temperature distribution may indicate underlying disease.

Heat lamp n=10 c=3 r=4,10

This is the infrared lamp used in the physiotherapy department for providing heat treatment to a stiff, painful or inflamed part of the body. Ultraviolet treatment lamps are sometimes wrongly described as heat lamps.

Because of the wavelengths delivered (770 to 12 000 nm), penetration is limited to 10 mm although the enhanced blood supply (due to the heat) may carry heat to deeper structures. The treatment regime might be a course of five treatment sessions during the recovery from an injury.

Such lamps are also used in the care and treatment of newborns who can be or must be removed from an enclosed incubator for examination and treatment.

Heat treatment unit r=4

Heat treatment is used extensively in the physiotherapy department for the relief of conditions such as pain, muscle spasm, stiffness and inflammation. Heat may be applied by conduction through the skin using a bath (water or wax), a hot pack (e.g. hydrocollator pack), or it may be applied remotely using electromagnetic radiation such as short waves, microwaves, infrared, or by ultrasound.

More information is given under the other headings.

Heated gloves/socks

These are used during the treatment of Raynaud's syndrome (White finger), chilblains, and arthritis. The basic system consists of knitted gloves with a fine heating element in the fingers and thumbs, or in the toe region in the case of heated socks. These are powered by a low-voltage rechargeable pack which is normally worn on the waist. A heated back-pack is also available which works on the same principle and is said to give some relief of back pain.

Heated ripple mattress n=10 c=3

These are used in intensive care and also sometimes in the operating theatre to provide heat, and protection against pressure sores. The mattress is normally a double sheet of plastic welded together to provide two separate channels for water to pass through. The so-called ripple effect is achieved by directing warm water through one channel for a few minutes, and then through the other so that the patient is supported on different parts of the mattress in the two phases of the cycle, thus avoiding prolonged pressure on any point on the body.

Typical parameters for a ripple heat mattress and controller might be heating from 20 to 37°C in 15 minutes from a 2 litre reservoir tank, a flow rate of 45 l/h in the ripple mode and twice this in the non-ripple mode. The ripple cycle might be 6 minutes.

Heating bath n=20 c=2,3

This is a small tank containing oil, water or wax, with a heater and thermostatic controller to achieve steady temperature in the fluid in the tank. The most common types are blood warmers in which water is heated to just above normal body temperature, through which blood is passed within a coil of plastic tubing, to raise its temperature to a suitable level before infusion into the body. In this case the bath consists of a stainless steel tank, an electric heater, a thermostat, and a stirrer to ensure even distribution of heat. The device usually has secondary overlimit temperature cut-out to operate in case of failure of the thermostat.

Heating baths containing oil are used in the pathology laboratory for raising the temperature of fluids undergoing chemical reactions. Similar baths containing wax are used in the physiotherapy department for imparting heat to diseased or injured limbs at just above body temperature. Heated wax baths are also used in the preparation of ear moulds for hearing aids.

Heidbrink valve n=200 c=1 r=2

This is an expiratory valve used in anaesthetic breathing circuits. Its purpose is to allow expired gases to pass out of the breathing circuit and to prevent outside air being drawn in during inspiration. It usually consists of a wide-bore T-tube suitable for inclusion in the breathing circuit close to the patient with the side arm containing a poppet valve in which the poppet is held against a collar by a light spring. The spring tension, and hence the opening pressure, is controlled by screwing down the valve top. When the valve top is screwed home the valve is locked closed. The valve is usually of metal construction and can be easily dismantled for cleaning or sterilizing.

Helium dilution (FRC) analyser n=1 c=4,5 r=3

The functional residual capacity (FRC) of the lungs can be found by diluting the gases in a rebreathing circuit with helium. The rebreathing circuit includes a spirometer, a CO_2 and water absorber and a fresh gas supply of oxygen at about 300 ml/min. A known quantity of helium is injected into the circuit and after a few breaths when helium has mixed with gases in all parts of the circuit and lungs, the concentration of helium is measured in a sample of the gas. The total volume of the closed circuit can then be easily calculated. The system is used in the lung function laboratory.

The helium analyser is usually based on the thermal conductivity of the gas. Since the sensor is not specific to helium a correction must be applied using a knowledge of the other gases in the mixture. Alternatively, the FRC may be calculated using a radioactive gas sample.

Heparin pump n=20 c=2,3 r=3

There is a tendency for blood to clot after passing through mechanical devices or when it comes into contact with synthetic materials. Thus an anticoagulant is required whenever blood is removed from the body.

The most commonly used anticoagulant is heparin, which is used in haemodialysis. The heparin pump, which may be a motorized syringe or a peristaltic roller pump, is employed to inject heparin into blood leaving the body before passing through the artificial kidney (dialyser), although it may sometimes be injected after the dialyser. The heparin is normally injected after the blood pump, since the pressure of the blood will always be positive at this point and the possibility of drawing in air through leaks is therefore eliminated.

Heparin pumps are also employed as part of heart–lung pumping procedures.

His bundle analyser n=1 c=4 r=3

The bundle of His (pronounced 'hiss') is a nerve trunk connecting the atrioventricular (AV) node in the heart to the main muscles and Purkinje fibres of the ventricles. A His bundle electrocardiogram (HBE) would show the point in time at which the AV node was first stimulated, and the point at which it in turn stimulates the His bundle, and then the contraction of the ventricles. In electronic terms the sequence of events from the natural pacemaker in the heart (the sinoatrial (SA) node) is like an astable multivibrator, followed by a delay line to the AV node which acts as a monostable delay mechanism to trigger the His bundle which again acts as a delay line feeding the signals to the muscles. The timing of these events is important to cause the upper and lower chambers of the heart to contract in the correct sequence.

Transmission along the His bundle may be defective in some cases, and it is possible to trace the path of the signal using a special-purpose analyser. Basically this consists of a stimulating probe and a pick-up probe by which a small pulse of electric current can be presented to the bundle through its surface and this can be detected at more distant points of the bundle. The presence of and timing of the arrival of the transmitted pulse are displayed and used to assess the extent and location of the defect.

Since the bundle of His is only accessible during cardiac surgery, this is a rather specialized device only likely to be used in heart surgery.

Hot pack heater $n=1$ $c=3$

In the physiotherapy department heat treatment is applied by various methods, one of which is a simple moist pack containing a gel. The packs are placed in a heated bath where they absorb up to ten times their weight of water, and are then taken out and applied to the skin under towels.

The hot pack heater is a simple thermostatically controlled water bath with special racking for holding the hot packs.

Humidifier $n=50$ $c=2$ $r=2$

During anaesthesia or artificial ventilation the body's natural humidification processes are often bypassed, with the result that there is a drying out of the trachea and larger bronchi. Humidifiers can be classified as follows:

1. Passive humidifiers such as the 'artificial nose'
2. True water vapour humidifiers, or nebulizers producing droplets of water
3. Hot or cold humidifiers
4. Those intended for humidifying the atmosphere or those intended for connection to an airway.

The mechanism of humidification may involve bubbling the gases through a bottle of water, or the use of a wick, atomizer, ultrasound, or hot water.

The temperature of the delivered gases and their handling on the way to the patient is most important since 100% relative humidity at room temperature may fall to 30% when the gases have been warmed in the lungs. With nebulizers the drop size is important since large drops will only serve to waterlog the lungs without the moisture reaching the alveoli.

Hydrocollator pack $r=4,10$

Amongst the large variety of methods of applying heat as a treatment for pain, muscle spasm, stiffness or inflammation, one method includes the application of hot packs against the skin, causing heating to a depth of 5 mm or so. Blood flow secondary to heat itself may carry energy to deeper structures. The hydrocollator pack is a canvas bag containing a silicone gel paste which absorbs an amount of water equal to ten times its weight. These are placed in water at 180°F and following absorption they can be used for 20 minutes. Special heating baths are also available.

Hydrotherapy apparatus n=1 c=5

This is a medical form of jacuzzi, being a heated bath in which the patient lies, and pulsating aerated water is jetted on to various parts of the body. This is claimed to be helpful in treating circulatory troubles, paralysis, nervous congestion, and also after burns, frost bite, etc. It usually has controls for temperature, and for the directing of the water jets on to various parts of the body. A simpler form of this is the whirlpool bath.

Hyfrecator n=3 c=2,3

This is a low-power surgical diathermy apparatus intended for the removal of warts, treatment of cervical erosion, excision of skin flaps, and in chiropody. Typical specifications are power output between 1 and 30 W. See also Surgical diathermy.

Hyperbaric therapy apparatus r=4

For treating respiratory insufficiency due to inadequate ventilation or circulatory problems, the patient may be totally enclosed in a pressure chamber in which the oxygen tension may be raised to provide useful amounts of oxygen in the blood through the respiratory system and through the skin. Larger units may allow the therapist to work in the chamber at the same time.

Hyperbaric chambers are also used in the re-acclimatization of deep-sea divers to atmospheric pressure.

Image intensifier r=7

This is an integral part of any diagnostic X-ray set which can produce a fluoroscopic image on a video monitor, or on cine film. X-rays can cause a fluorescent screen to glow in the form of the X-ray image, and early fluoroscopes employed this principle to provide moving pictures which had to be viewed in total darkness.

The image intensifier enhances the brightness of the image many times (e.g. ×1000 to ×5000) so that it can be televised or filmed for daylight viewing. The image intensifier itself is an electronic device contained in a large evacuated glass envelope. It comprises a fluorescent screen on to which the X-rays fall, and this is in contact with a second layer (photocathode) which emits electrons in response to light from the fluorescent screen. The rest of the image intensifier is an electron accelerator and focusing system which produces a smaller brighter image on a second phosphorescent screen similar to a CRT screen. The image on this second screen can be viewed by the cine or video camera.

Fluoroscopic (or screening) systems using image intensifiers are useful for a large number of examinations for which a moving image is essential. Unfortunately they cannot match the sharpness of detail obtained with conventional X-ray film and cassettes.

Impedance bridge n=1 c=3

An electronic impedance bridge is a device for calculating the impedance of an unknown resistor, capacitor or inductor (or combination of these), usually employing the Wheatstone bridge principle. Such units would only be found in an electronics laboratory in a hospital. The term impedance bridge may also be found in connection with the acoustic impedance (or admittance) bridge used in audiology clinics to assess middle ear pressure and other characteristics of the middle ear.

Electrical impedance measurements may also be used to replace a mercury-in-rubber strain gauge during venous occlusion plethysmography.

Impedance plethysmograph n=1 c=4 r=3

The electrical impedance between two electrodes placed on the skin surface will vary in response to volume changes in the tissue between them. Electrodes placed at two points down the leg will record electrical impedance which will vary in time with arterial pulsations, and similarly, electrodes on the chest can be used to sense changes in resistance caused by different blood volumes in the chest at various parts of the cardiac cycle. Changes in volume due to breathing can also be detected.

The resistance is normally sensed using alternating currents between 1 and 100 kHz, with a constant current drive of (say) 100 μA. The impedance measurements may be made by two- or four-electrode techniques. The four-electrode technique partially eliminates electrode-skin impedance problems.

Electrical impedance plethysmography has a number of theoretical problems in application, but its most important areas of potential use (cardiac output estimation and peripheral blood flow) are alternatives to invasive and dangerous procedures. It seems likely therefore that the development of the subject will continue until the technique is sufficiently reliable to replace some of these other techniques.

Such devices might be found in the cardiology department or in the vascular surgery unit.

Incubator n=10 c=4 r=4,6

This may be a piece of laboratory apparatus used for keeping fluids at approximately blood temperature to speed up a chemical or biological reaction, or it may be a temperature-controlled chamber for a premature baby. In the case of the premature baby the natural temperature control mechanism is inadequately developed and so it must be cared for in the early weeks of its life in a special chamber.

The infant incubator is normally in the form of a trolley with a small mattress in the top covered by a rigid clear plastic cover which may be removed to nurse the baby or may have closable ports in the cover through which the nurse's hands may be passed. Underneath the baby is an air-blown electric heating system which circulates air at about 33°C through the incubator chamber. The temperature control may be a thermostat in the heated air stream, a thermistor and electronic control, or a temperature sensor may be placed on the abdomen of the baby.

While the baby is being nursed in the incubator, extra oxygen may be introduced into the air in the chamber, or the infant may be artificially ventilated. It is also common to monitor the breathing pattern of the baby, particularly to identify episodes of non-breathing (apnoea), and the skin oxygen tension may also be monitored using a tiny polarographic cell on the skin. Transcutaneous oxygen tension monitoring works relatively well in neonates compared with adults because the skin is more permeable to gases.

Each hospital caring for newborn babies also needs to have at least one transport incubator which is lighter than the conventional models and can be run for a few hours on battery power. These are required for transporting babies between hospitals. This is quite common since not every maternity unit will have the facilities to care for premature, or very small babies.

Indifferent electrode r=4

During monopolar electrosurgery metal plates with large surface area (e.g. 100 cm^2) are used to draw off the current applied for cutting or coagulation by the active electrode. These are flexible plates applied on the buttocks or around the leg of patients undergoing surgery, and are required to achieve a low impedance contact with the skin. This may be achieved by a leg electrode enveloped in cloth soaked in saline, or jelly may be used between the electrode and the skin. Capacitance coupling may also be employed, using electrodes covered with a thin plastic film. A constant worry during electrosurgery is that the indifferent or dispersive electrode may be making poor contact with the skin, or that the lead to it may be disconnected or fractured. One of these problems may be overcome by the use of a fault detection device (often called a Flexoplate monitor) which verifies a conductive contact between the electrosurgery unit and the indifferent plate.

Inductive loop

This term refers to a communication system, either for staff paging or as a hearing aid, in which a loop of wire surrounds the area to be covered. Receivers within the loop respond to a low-frequency carrier current passing around the loop on which the calling codes or speech is superimposed.

A number of types of hearing aid can be switched to bypass the internal microphone and instead receive the signals directly from the inductive loop system. This has proved particularly useful in providing amplified speech without the complication of room acoustics and other noises close to the listener. Such systems are often installed in schools where deaf children are taught, and in some cases the range may extend to the sports fields.

A number of systems in use actually employ VHF radio transmission but are still (wrongly) called inductive loop systems.

Inductothermy apparatus r=4

Deep heating of body tissues as a treatment for pain, spasm, stiffness and inflammation, as applied in the physiotherapy department, may include short-wave diathermy which causes heating of the tissues with higher electrolyte content in response to electromagnetic radiation passed through the body.

The frequency employed is usually 27 MHz, applied by placing two large insulated metal electrodes, one each side of the region to be treated. The tissue acts as the dielectric in a capacitor, and heat is liberated due to the dielectric loss. The same effect can be brought about using a spiral or helix of wire to produce an oscillating magnetic field within the body which will induce currents having the same effect. This is called inductothermy and may be used to apply heating on a single flat surface where the two electrode approach would not be possible. Sometimes the effect is produced by winding an insulated wire around the limb being treated. The flat inductive 'pancake' coil produces heating up to 40 mm below the skin.

Infrared camera

This device provides a picture of the patient or part of a patient using infrared radiation from the skin which relates closely to a surface temperature map. The topic is covered more fully in Heat camera.

Infrared carbon dioxide analyser $n=1$ $c=4$ $r=9$

Gases may be identified by the extent to which they absorb infrared light. Instruments are available which utilize this property to estimate carbon dioxide content in breathing gases, but other gases may also be identified. This is a type of absorption spectrometer.

Infrared radiation is passed through two parallel chambers to a detection device (usually a Golay or Luft cell) which records the difference in infrared absorption in the two chambers. A chopping disc causes the infrared light to pass through each chamber in turn causing alternating displacement of a diaphragm in the Golay cell. The diaphragm will be displaced to one side or other depending on the relative quantities of infrared light reaching the absorption chambers. An electronic circuit used to amplify, demodulate and linearize the output is connected to the capacitance displacement transducer attached to the diaphragm.

One of the chambers is filled with a reference gas while the other is filled with a background gas plus a small flow-through of the gas being sampled. The modification in absorption is used to detect the molar fraction of the sample gases. Problems arise where the absorption spectra of the gases being tested overlap (e.g. nitrous oxide and halothane, carbon dioxide and carbon monoxide). The device requires a long stabilization period and the results will be affected by changes in atmospheric pressure.

Such instruments can be used for the analysis of gases in the lung function laboratory, and in the metabolic computer used in the intensive care department.

Infrared lamp n=5 c=3 r=4

Heat is widely employed in the physiotherapy department for treating pain, muscle spasm, stiffness and inflammation. The source of heat employed depends upon the depth of penetration required. Infrared radiation may be used where penetration is not required beyond 10 mm and employs wavelengths between 770 and 12 000 nm. The lamps are placed above the patient or affected area and kept on for the prescribed treatment period.

The lamp used may emit visible light or not. Those not emitting visible light are often called radiant heat sources, and employ wound or enclosed elements similar to those used in domestic electric heaters. Those producing visible light are usually tungsten filament lamps with a filter to reduce visible and ultraviolet radiation. They may be arranged singly or in arrays as in the tunnel bath.

Infrared lamps and radiant heat sources are also used in the care of small babies where they do not need an enclosed warm environment or are removed from an incubator for examination and treatment. In this case the heat lamps are arranged over the cot in which the baby lies.

Infrared viewer n=1 c=3

One of the standard tests in the investigation of dizziness or vertigo involves asking the patient to look in different directions while the clinician observes the patient's eyes in order to detect an abnormal eye movement called nystagmus. In the normal clinical environment, only patients with acute vestibular problems will exhibit this particular symptom since their eyes will be held steady by observation of the surroundings. A much more sensitive test is to do this in darkness, and there are several methods by which the patient's eye movement can be detected. The best method of achieving this is to use an electro-nystagmograph although an infrared viewer or Frenzel glasses also allow a subjective assessment of eye movement.

An infrared viewer is a hand-held battery-powered device which contains an infrared light source (which is invisible) to illuminate the patient's eyes. The reflected light is passed through an optical system containing a non-linear optical cell having the effect of doubling the frequency of the light, which brings the light into the visible spectrum to provide a monochromatic image (usually an eerie green).

Horizontal and vertical nystagmus can be readily observed with this method although true rotary nystagmus (where the eyes rotate about their

145

axis of view) is very difficult to detect. The device uses technology developed for the night sights used on rifles.

Infusion controller n=20 n=2,3

Instead of using a pump to deliver intravenous fluids in exact quantities or at precise flow rates, a simpler device may be used which only monitors the quantity and rate of fluid being infused. It usually works by counting the number or rate of drops passing through the drip chamber on the standard giving set (drip-set), and using this signal to operate a gate to stop and start the flow process. This type of controller has the advantage that the pressure applied cannot be greater than the head of the reservoir bag or bottle and so air is unlikely to be passed into the patient since there is no motive force once the infusion source is exhausted.

Infusion pump n=100 c=2,3,4 r=4

Infusion pumps and controllers are used extensively for delivering intravenous fluids and drugs as part of the care of patients in hospital. These are usually pumps but the term is often used loosely to describe an infusion controller which relies on the head of the fluid reservoir for its motive force, and merely controls the rate at which the fluid is dispensed.

Infusion pumps may be motorized syringes used for the slow delivery of small quantities of fluid or drugs or they may operate from a reservoir bag pumping and regulating the rate of passage of fluid along the giving set.

There are two main types which work from a reservoir. There are those which pump by applying peristaltic pressures to the outside of the giving set and measure the rate of flow by counting the drops passing through an optical gate clipped on to the drip chamber. Other types employ a disposable double syringe unit (cassette) connected into the giving set which draws in measured quantities of fluid according to the required infusion rate, and simultaneously dispenses from the other side of the syringe plunger. These are usually called volumetric pumps.

The drop-counting infusion pumps and controllers may produce erroneous rates of infusion if the drop-counting mechanism is confused by incorrect placement or extraneous light input. Most modern pumps have adequate protection circuitry and alarms to prevent the common hazards, but operator problems are still common. The so-called volumetric pumps employing the bi-directional syringe units (cassettes) involve relatively high costs for the disposable cassettes but are more reliable and accurate. Basic syringe pumps may cause trouble if unsuitable syringes are used, or if they must work against a high back pressure. Small battery operated and clockwork types exist which can be carried on the person where long-term infusion at very slow flow rates is required.

146

Injector suction unit n=300 c=1 r=2

Suction for aspiration of body fluids may be provided from a compressed gas supply (pipeline or cylinder) by the use of an injector or venturi. Depending on the design, it may provide high suction or high displacement. When driven from an oxygen cylinder they are wasteful of oxygen but have the advantage of portability. Such units are sometimes found in wards in hospitals and consist of the injector unit, which may plug into the piped gas supply, a reservoir bottle for the fluids and a suction catheter with suction nozzle. They are useful for short term use.

Ink-jet recorder n=2 c=4

One method of producing graphical records of rapidly changing signals (e.g. electromyographs) is by the use of a penless recorder in which ink is sprayed in a narrow jet from the axis of a galvanometer. Such recorders can produce a frequency response up to 1000 Hz since the inertia of the writing device is so small.

Insufflation apparatus n=5 c=3,4

This delivers carbon dioxide under low pressure to open up a space within the body. Its most common application is in endoscopy through flexible or rigid endoscopes to give a sufficiently large viewing area. An example is in laparoscopy when the viewing instrument is passed through a small incision in the abdomen. A space is created by carbon dioxide insufflation for viewing and internal surgery. Insufflation has also been used in the uterus to diagnose and treat blocked fallopian tubes.

Carbon dioxide is used since it will be readily absorbed into the tissues after the procedure. The apparatus normally consists of a carbon dioxide cylinder, a regulator to reduce the pressure, and a small rotameter flowmeter and needle valve to control the rate of flow. Sometimes a pressure gauge and relief valve are included. Such devices are commonly found in operating theatres.

Integrator r=9

This is basically an electronic circuit for calculating the product of input voltage and time. A steady input voltage will produce a slowly rising ramp of output, whereas a short pulse will cause a small rise with no further change until there is new input. Integrators are employed in electromyography (EMG) equipment to produce a voltage which will represent the electromyographic activity. The EMG signal is first rectified and then fed to the

147

integrator. The integrator will of course reach a saturation voltage after a time and the usual way of dealing with this is to reset the integrator to zero and present a pulse on a separate recording channel or to a counter which will indicate the total activity which has occurred during the test procedure.

Integrating circuits are often used with a leak resistor to discharge the capacitor at a known rate. This is no longer a true integrator but an exponential averager as used in some cardiotachometers and other pulse rate meters.

Interferential treatment unit n=3 c=4 r=10

Electrotherapy and faradic treatment of muscle pain, strains, and oedema are sometimes ineffective at treating sites deep within the body because the electrical current required is restricted by the high impedance at the skin electrodes. Electrical impedance at the skin reduces rapidly as the frequency is increased but so does the therapeutic effect. A differential treatment system employs two medium frequency (e.g. 4000 Hz and 4010 Hz) stimulating currents fed through skin electrodes at the opposite corners of a square so that they interfere where they cross over at the centre of the square. A stimulating current at the beat frequency (the numerical difference between the stimulating frequencies) is produced in the treatment region.

A low beat frequency of, say, 10 Hz may be generated for the the treatment of muscle disorders, and a higher frequency (e.g. 100 Hz) generated for the relief of pain.

Such apparatus is used in the physiotherapy department, often in conjunction with suction electrodes which may also provide a therapeutic 'suction massage'.

Intermittent blower ventilator n=6 c=4 r=2

These are lung ventilators driven by a continuous flow of gases or air, usually at a pressure of 45 to 60 psi. Only a part of the driving gas is delivered to the patient and other gases may be added by means of an injector. They are most commonly used for intensive care rather than anaesthesia. Examples are the Bird ventilators and the Cyclator.

Intermittent compression apparatus n=5 c=3

A range of inflatable appliances, which apply intermittent compression to various parts of the body, have been developed. Perhaps the best known of these are the inflatable leggings which are used for the prevention of deep vein thrombosis during immobilization. The principle here is to inflate the appliance two or three times a minute to move blood out of the limb.

A number of other similar devices exist which fit on other parts of the body and are used to encourage fluid transfer in cases of oedema, leg ulcers, etc. The same technique and instrumentation is also used to provide physiotherapy in some muscle disorders.

The inflatable appliance may be almost any shape or size to fit the patient and part of the body being treated, but the pulsating pump is common to a number of applications and typically includes an air pump, pressure gauge and controls to select treatment time, and the frequency and intensity of pressure pulsations. Some devices can be linked to faradic treatment units so that the pressure cycles are synchronized with pulsations in the electrical treatment.

Intermittent flow apparatus $n=10$ $c=4$ $r=2$

An intermittent flow or demand flow apparatus is a type of anaesthetic/ analgesic machine in which gases only flow in response to the patient's respiratory effort. These are often portable and are used for dental anaesthesia, emergency surgery, and for analgesia during labour. All the common types are designed to deliver a mixture of nitrous oxide and oxygen, although some can be used with vaporizers, but these must be low-resistance types (draw-over vaporizers). The basic principle of demand flow apparatus is that cylinders of high-pressure gas fill one or more reservoirs (bags or bellows) at low pressure via pressure reducing valves. The reservoir (or mixing chamber in the case of variable mixture machines) is connected to the breathing circuit via a light valve which opens under the slight negative pressure created when the patient attempts to breath in. During expiration the reservoirs refill.

The simplest form of intermittent flow apparatus uses premixed gases such as in the Entonox apparatus; most others include a mechanism for mixing the gases. Examples of mixing valve types are the Mckesson, Lucy Baldwyn, Walton 5, AE, and Quantiflex RA. Some of these can also deliver a continuous flow of the mixed gases and include features found on other anaesthetic machines, such as oxygen flush and rotameter flowmeters.

Intermittent positive pressure ventilator (IPPV) $n=30$ $c=4$ $r=2$

This is the most common form of ventilator used during anaesthesia or in intensive care (life support) to assist or replace the patient's own respiratory effort. It consists of a mechanism for inflating the lungs in a rhythmic pattern, usually via a cuffed tube inserted into the trachea. This is sometimes called a lung ventilator, or is referred to by some feature of its operation (e.g. minutes volume divider).

149

It consists of a breathing circuit containing bellows, bags, tubes, valves, filters, and measuring transducers, and a drive and control circuit including timing devices, motors, solenoids and valves. There are a large number of variations on the main theme, a few of which are given below.

1. Application – whether it is to be used during anaesthesia, or for intensive care. Some types cannot be used for both.
2. Breathing circuit – whether suitable for use in closed, open, or T-piece circuits.
3. Driving force – whether driven by electric motor, compressed gas, or from a continuous flow anaesthetic machine.
4. Type of ventilation – main types include constant pressure, volume, or flow.
5. Method of cycle timing – this may be by time, preset volume, pressure, or triggered by the patient.
6. Respiratory pattern – particular machines may be able to vary the relative lengths of the phases and be able to provide positive, atmospheric, or negative pressure during all or part of the expiratory phase.
7. Other features which may need specification when selecting an automatic IPPV for a specific job are the peak inspiratory flow rate, flexibility of performance, ease of sterilization, portability, and suitability for particular patients such as infants, or those with low compliance lungs.

Intra-aortic balloon r=4

This is the active element in a complex device for assisting the performance of the heart in chronic failure or during a weaning phase after cardiopulmonary bypass.

A smooth polyurethane balloon, several centimetres in length, is passed into the descending aorta through the femoral artery. The balloon is rapidly inflated during early diastole, and deflated in early systole, synchronized by the ECG signal. Inflation during diastole augments arterial and coronary perfusion pressure, and deflation during systole reduces aortic impedance to ventricular ejection, thus relieving the heart of some of its load.

Although simple in concept, the exact control required over the timing and extent of inflation presents problems and requires specially trained operators. A more complex balloon design may be used to reduce the abnormally high pressures which are caused in the proximal segment of the aorta. In this case the balloon has several compartments fed by orifices of different diameter to cause the sequential inflation of the different segments of the balloon. The inflating gas may be helium or carbon dioxide, but helium is safer since it will diffuse quickly through the arterial wall in the case of leakage, and is inert. Carbon dioxide released into the blood increases the acidity.

The intra-aortic balloon may be used continuously for several months or operate intermittently. Clotting may occur if the deflated balloon remains in the aorta for any length of time and manual operation may be necessary if arrhythmias prevent automatic triggering.

Ion selective electrode r=5

Measurement of the concentration of specific ions in solutions (both *in vivo* and *in vitro*) can be made by selective electrodes. Examples are hydrogen (pH), chloride, potassium, sodium, calcium, etc.

There are two main types. Direct measurement electrodes measure the activity or concentration of an ion in water or plasma. Indirect types measure the activity or concentration in a dilution of the original sample. The direct measurement types are independent of the effects of abnormal levels of lipids or plasma proteins, and can be used with whole blood.

Ionization chamber n=5 c=1 r=3

Ionizing radiation can be detected by the small electric current which can be made to flow between two electrodes when particles of the gas between them become ionized. The electrodes and gas are often in a sealed glass envelope to allow the gas pressure to be reduced, which makes the device more sensitive. The Geiger-Müller (GM) tube is a special type of ionization chamber which contains low-pressure neon or argon, and a very high voltage is applied between specially shaped electrodes. Ionization chambers are used to measure X-ray and gamma-ray radiation levels.

Small radiation monitors employing ionization chambers are available for personal dose monitoring, and GM tube instruments are available with a dose rate alarm. However, these instruments are not suitable for monitoring the dose rate to large numbers of individuals and so film badge monitors or thermoluminescent dosimetry devices are used.

Ionizing radiation r=3,4

Electromagnetic and particulate radiations may have sufficient energy to remove electrons from atoms (ionization). The energy of electromagnetic radiation is related to the frequency (or wavelength). Ionization of some atoms begins with rays of about 10 eV which corresponds to waves in the ultraviolet region. Thus visible light (1 eV), microwaves (0.0001 eV) and lower frequencies may be considered to be non-ionizing.

Ionization in human tissues is caused deliberately in radiotherapy using X-rays (0.1–10 MeV) and gamma rays (up to 100 MeV). Particulate

151

radiations of beta particles (electrons), alpha particles, neutrons, and heavy nuclei may also be used.

Iontophoresis apparatus r=4

This usually refers to the application of drugs through the skin as a result of positive ion transport caused by passing an electric current into the body. The apparatus required is a direct current generator of a few microamperes, and the drug is often a specially prepared hydrocortisone solution, applied under the positive electrode. In this example, pain and inflammation are reduced simultaneously.

The same principle has also been applied to the stimulating of sweat production for chemical analysis.

Iron lung n=0 c=4 r=2

This is an early type of breathing machine (ventilator) now almost fallen into disuse. The patient is placed in a cabinet sealed at the neck leaving only the head outside. The pressure in the cabinet is cycled so that the chest is forced to expand and contract with the pressure in the cabinet, so ventilating the lungs. These were relatively inefficient. Air would also be drawn into the stomach, nursing was extremely difficult, and the seal at the neck difficult to maintain.

Isolating transformer n=5 c=1 r=2

The mains electricity supply has a neutral conductor which is in fact earthed at the local substation, and a live conductor which is approximately 250 V above earth (in Europe). This presents a hazard during accidental contact with the live conductor if a route to earth is provided through the body. A partial solution to this problem can be provided for situations where equipment must be opened while connected to the mains by the inclusion of an isolating transformer in the mains supply. This creates a new mains supply which has neither conductor connected to earth so that risk of electrocution only occurs if both conductors are touched simultaneously. The transformer has two identical but isolated windings.

Isolating transformers are often used on benches where electrical or electronic equipment is serviced. They are less used now since the introduction of earth leakage circuit breakers (ELCBs) or residual current circuit breakers (RCCBs) which detect the difference in current in the two supply leads and disconnect the supply if this exceeds preset limits.

Isolette negative pressure apparatus r=4

This is a whole-body 'iron lung' type of ventilator for infants which works by creating a negative pressure around the thorax to cause inspiration to the lungs.

Isotope cow n=1 r=3

This is an old name for a radionuclide generator, for the continuous production of short-life radioactive isotopes (radionuclides). An arrangement in common use in hospitals (in the medical physics or nuclear medicine department) is a column containing molybdenum-99 as ammonium molybdate. This continually produces technetium-99m, which has a short half-life (6 hours) and is much used in nuclear medicine. The technetium can be flushed out of the column with saline, and appears as sodium pertechnetate.

Isotope scanner n=6 c=5,6 r=3

This normally refers to a rectilinear scanner for producing a map of the sites of radioactivity within a particular organ. The isotopes (radionuclides) are usually administered attached to a chemical (radiopharmaceutical) that is absorbed or used by the organ under study (e.g. thyroid, liver, blood, bone). The scanner uses a scintillation counter to map the extent of uptake of the agent. They are used in the nuclear medicine or X-ray department.

J

Jackson Rees paediatric T-tube c=1 r=2

A paediatric endotracheal tube which has an integral T-piece which is useful in non-rebreathing anaesthetic circuits not employing valves (which cause back pressure). It also has a stoppered connection in line with the tube which provides a facility for suction.

K

Katharometer n=2 c=3 r=9

This is a thermal conductivity detector for gases employing heated wires which are cooled by the gases to be identified. In general the thermal conductivity of a gas is inversely related to its molecular weight. Hydrogen and helium, for example, have conductivities approximately 6.5 times those of nitrogen and oxygen. The katharometer normally consists of two parallel tubes in which are mounted heating elements arranged in a bridge circuit so that resistance changes due to unequal cooling by the gases in each tube can be detected. One channel normally receives a reference gas (e.g. helium) and the gas mixture to be analysed is passed through the other.

Katharometers are used in lung function testing equipment such as the helium FRC analyser, and in the gas chromatograph. Response times are poor (e.g. 10 seconds to 1 minute) compared with a mass spectrometer, but the cost is low and accuracy can be high.

Kromayer lamp r=10

This is a water-cooled mercury-vapour lamp producing high-intensity ultraviolet radiation for physiotherapy. Its special feature is that it can be applied directly to the area to be treated. It is water cooled and the rays actually pass through the water to remove infrared radiation.

kV$_p$ meter n=1 c=3,4

The energy distribution of the output of a diagnostic X-ray set is determined by the type of tube in use and also by the kilovoltage applied to that tube.

The peak kilovoltage (kV$_p$) can be measured by direct electrical connection to an X-ray tube circuit using a voltage divider circuit, or alternatively it can be determined indirectly from the X-ray beam. Devices for indirect determination of kV$_p$ usually employ the known attenuation of different X-ray energies through copper sheeting. The different X-ray intensities perceived on the upper and lower side of a copper sheet can be detected and delivered to a computing circuit to calculate the originating kilovoltage.

Such devices may be used by the X-ray service engineer, or in the X-ray

155

department as part of a quality assurance programme for verifying the consistent performance of the X-ray set.

Kymograph

Literally this means a wave-writer, and so the term could be applied to almost any form of chart recorder. The term is most commonly used to mean a simple form of chart recorder having a rotating drum around which the recording paper is wrapped and the writing pen moves along the length of the drum as the input signal changes. These are rather old-fashioned instruments, often driven by clockwork, and in some cases the outside of the drum is blackened with soot instead of using recording paper. The recording stylus then scribes a visible line in the soot. Kymographs are still found from time to time in hospital equipment such as spirometers in which a simple mechanical linkage between the breath-sensing cylinder or bellows can operate the recording pen without the need for electronics.

L

Laryngograph n=1 c=3,4

This measures electrical impedance through the larynx during sound production (phonation), providing an electrical waveform which can be displayed on a cathode ray tube. The waveform can be examined for normal, falsetto, creaky, and pathological patterns, and can also show frequency changes. Two electrodes are applied superficially to the neck while the patient speaks. Such devices are used in the speech therapy department.

An alternative name for this instrument is the electroglottograph, and an extended version including a display of the speech fundamental frequency is called a voiscope.

Laryngoscope n=50 c=1 r=2

This is a hand-held lever and light used for depressing the tongue and viewing prior to insertion of an artificial airway. The commonest type is the Mackintosh curved folding airway. There are also Magill laryngoscopes. A range of sizes is available, and the batteries are normally in the handle. The handle can be separated from the 'blade' for cleaning and sterilizing.

Laser (surgical) n=2 c=6 r=4,9

A focused beam of laser light may be used for cutting and coagulating tissue with great precision without the probe needing to touch the tissue. Laser light can be focused to achieve great intensity (e.g. 10 kW/cm^2) on to very tiny points.

Perhaps the best known application is the photocoagulation of points on the retina of the eye using the argon laser. The light beam may be directed through the cornea on to the retina using the natural focusing system of the eye under the full view of the surgeon. Bleeding points on the retina can be coagulated and re-attachment of the retina can be achieved. The area of the coagulation can be as small as 10 μm in diameter and the short time of application allows very little spread of the heat to the surrounding tissue. Garnet crystal lasers (Nb:YAG) are also used.

The carbon dioxide laser is now finding application in surgery and this produces light in the infrared region. Unfortunately these wavelengths cannot be conveyed through optic fibres and so must be reflected through the manipulating arm by a series of mirrors and lenses which are opaque to visible light (germanium lenses are often used). Laser light is normally absorbed and converted into heat in the first millimetre or so of tissue and so their application is for the cutting or coagulation of surface lesions without damage to deeper structures. Since the light will be absorbed in any surface water or exudate, a gas jet or flushing system is often employed to clear any liquid away.

Leakage current monitor

Small electric currents from mains-powered apparatus may unintentionally pass through the patient. Since these currents are normally very small they are not perceived by the hospital staff. There has been considerable attention paid to assessing the magnitudes of these currents which may be hazardous in patients, and to ensuring that equipment items do not individually or collectively deliver dangerous levels of leakage current, even when the equipment is faulty. For further information see Earth leakage current monitor.

Light beam diaphragm $r=7$

In diagnostic X-ray examination it is important to restrict the radiation to the smallest possible area, and therefore a localizing cone or diaphragm is used. In most X-ray sets there is a lamp and suitable optical mechanisms to allow projection on to the patient of the area to be irradiated. The diaphragm is then adjusted to cover only the area to be examined before the X-ray system is actuated. This mechanism is known as a light beam diaphragm.

Light pen $r=1$

Instructions may be given to a computer by the use of a light pen. This is a hand-held probe which has a light detector at its tip which is connected to the computer. If the pen is held to the face of the visual display unit the position on the screen is known to the computer by the time at which the light pen receives the pulse of light from the scanning spot as it passes underneath it. Depending on the type of computer program it is thus possible to enter graphical information into the computer or answer questions by touching particular spots on the display.

Light pens are now sometimes used with ultrasonic B-scanners and with some nuclear medicine imaging apparatus to draw round a particular organ or region of interest seen on the display. Such images of the body are normally held in a computer memory (e.g. digital scan converter) and so are

158

readily accessible to this type of computer input. A typical application might be drawing a line around the circumference of the foetal trunk as seen on an ultrasonic B-scan. The computer program might then present a figure for the area contained, the estimated weight of the foetus, or its estimated maturity.

Light pens form an extremely fast and flexible form of computer input without the use of a keyboard.

Light plethysmograph n=1 c=2 r=3

The amount of light reflected from beneath the skin surface will depend on the volume of blood that is present, and this will vary in a pulsatile manner. In theory this technique could be used to give some quantitative information about the blood supply to the extremities in vascular disease. However, its commonest use is simply as a pulse monitor in the operating theatre or high dependency unit.

The whole plethysmograph simply consists of a sensing head which is placed on a finger tip or on the ear lobe and contains a light source and photocell. The light source is often a conventional tungsten bulb which will provide a little heat to improve the local blood circulation. The reflected light is picked up by a photocell, which is usually a photoresistor. The probe is connected to a detector unit which senses the light fluctuations and presents these on a meter, cathode ray tube, or rate-meter.

Linear accelerator n=1 c=5,6 r=3,4

Electrons can be accelerated to high velocities (up to 99% of the speed of light) in a straight wave guide driven by a microwave (e.g. 10 GHz) generator. Electrons are fed from a thermionic source into the evacuated wave guide which contains a series of metal diaphragms with a hole in the middle so that with each wave the electrons move from one diaphragm to the next. The spacing of the diaphragms is increased down the length of the tube as the velocity of the electrons increases. At the far end they strike an X-ray target from which high-energy X-rays (4–15 MeV) are produced, or pass through a window to allow direct electron treatment.

The resultant X-ray beam is attenuated by a beam-flattening filter, a circular piece of metal, thicker in the centre than at the edge, which is introduced into the beam to produce a uniform X-ray intensity. The beam size is controlled by metal shutters, usually adjustable over the range 4–30 cm. Beam intensity may be modified by a variety of metal filters, the commonest being wedge shaped, which attenuate uniformly from one side of the beam to the other.

Such devices are used in the radiotherapy department for the treatment of deep cancers since these high-energy rays have good penetration properties.

The machine is designed so that the beam can be rotated about the patient to provide maximum dose to a point at the centre of rotation and less dose at all radial sites.

Linear array (ultrasound) scanner n=3 c=5,6 r=1

The most common type of moving picture ultrasonic scanner uses a linear array transducer. This is a large transducer which has a contact area with the skin of approximately 1 cm by 10 cm. Inside the transducer the piezoelectric element is divided into many parallel elements along the 10 cm length and these are connected by electronic switching so that only a small area (e.g. 1 cm by 1 cm) of the transducer is active at any time. With the active area at one end of the transducer an ultrasonic pulse is transmitted, and echoes are detected from the tissue immediately beneath this area. On the B-scan display this produces a line of bright dots. Then the active area commutates along the transducer repeating the process so that many parallel lines of scan are produced on the screen. The process is repeated so that the complete scan is refreshed on to the screen at greater than the flicker frequency of the eye, thus producing a moving picture.

Moving picture scans have a number of advantages particularly where there is rapid movement of the structures in the scanning plane (e.g. heart). The scan is a 'simple' scan in that each point in the tissue is interrogated from one direction only, so theoretically some information may be lost. However, the diagnostic information is usually greater than with the static B-scanners except where a large field of view is required or where the skin surface cannot be flattened to accommodate the large contact area.

Most modern scanners include a frame freeze module in which the level of brightness (echo amplitude) at every point on the picture is stored in a computer memory so that the motion of the picture can be arrested for examination or recording. A larger field of view can be generated by freezing adjacent areas of the image on some scanners.

The main ultrasonic generation and processing sections of the scanner are the same as for the basic A-scanner. The only necessary extra is the control circuitry to activate the selected areas of the multi-element transducer and relate this to the correct lines on the picture.

Linear variable differential transformer (LVDT) r=9

This is an inductive displacement transducer sometimes used in pressure, displacement and force transducers. Sensitivity for LVDTs is much higher than for strain gauges but the processing apparatus is more complex. There are various types but the commonest has a primary coil wound around a sliding metal core with a secondary winding around the two ends of the core.

As the core is displaced the voltage induced in the secondary winding changes such that the output voltage increases as the core moves to each side of the centre position and the phase changes by 180 degrees as it passes through the centre. A phase sensitive detector is required to convert the signal into a displacement. In pressure transducers the sliding core is connected to the pressure diaphragm.

Liquid oxygen supply n=1 c=7 r=2

A central piped medical gas supply is provided in larger hospitals for reasons of economy of scale. In the case of oxygen it can be provided more cheaply by the use of a liquid oxygen reservoir since larger quantities can be stored and delivered at one time. The oxygen is stored in an outside reservoir which can be filled without disconnecting the supply. The reserve is monitored on a force platform to estimate the weight of the remaining oxygen.

Some heating is required to bring the resulting gas up to a suitable temperature and it is usual to have a back-up supply of gaseous oxygen in cylinder banks. The maintenance of these (liquid) systems is normally performed by the suppliers.

Liquid scintillation counter n=2 c=6 r=3

Gamma rays of less than 20 keV and beta rays of less than 500 keV cannot be counted by the usual sodium iodide type of scintillation counter. This problem is overcome in the liquid scintillation counter (also known as a beta counter) by mixing the scintillator with the sample and using photomultiplier (PM) tubes to count the scintillations. The scintillators used are complex organic molecules, and secondary scintillators may be used to convert the wavelength to match the PM tube. The sample and PM tubes must be housed in a light-tight box.

The PM tube itself produces emission of electrons which may affect the results and so the sample is often cooled (e.g. to 5°C) and only scintillations detected simultaneously by two tubes are counted.

Normally several hundred samples are counted in turn by use of an automatic sample changer, and calibration and background samples are included, to enable computer correction factors to be included in the results.

These devices are intended for counting low-energy isotopes such as tritium and carbon 14. They may be found in chemical pathology, nuclear medicine, and immunology departments, used for radioimmunoassay (RIA), or competitive binding analysis.

Lithotriptor n=3 c=4,8

This is a stone breaker which may be required for the breaking and removal of stones in the kidney, ureter or bladder. Most lithotriptors are used in conjunction with endoscopes and employ remotely operated tools to grasp and break the stones. The fragments may in some cases be withdrawn through a suction channel in the endoscope. More advanced types employ ultrasonic shock waves to destroy the stones, and the shock wave may be delivered by a high-energy spark ignition at the tip of the operating endoscope or may generate mechanical vibration at the tip by an ultrasonic generator outside the body. A non-invasive type exists which generates a focused beam of ultrasound which is suitable for breaking stones within the kidney, which may remove the need for surgical intervention.

Load cell transducer

This is a force transducer used for measuring force or for weighing. It usually consists of a strain gauge transducer measuring the extension of a load element which has a known force/extension relationship. If high-frequency response is required piezoelectric types are used with a small crystal measuring the strain. In this case the electronic apparatus required in conjunction with the load cell is more complex. Other types of strain or displacement transducer may be used as part of the load cell.

Low-resistance vaporizer n=5 c=2 r=2

Where an anaesthetic vaporizer is required to fit into a closed breathing circuit or where the gases are drawn through it by the inspiratory effort of the patient it must have a low resistance to the passage of the gases. Examples are the Goldman Halothane vaporizer, the McKesson, and Rowbottom. Low-resistance vaporizers may sometimes be called 'draw-over' vaporizers.

Lung ventilator n=30 c=4 r=2,6

This is a machine for assisting breathing during anaesthesia or intensive care, which operates by applying intermittent positive pressure ventilation (IPPV) to the lungs via a tracheal tube which has an inflatable cuff to provide an airtight seal. Details of the types available may be found under Intermittent positive pressure ventilator.

M

M-mode (ultrasonic) scanner n=2 c=5,6 r=1

Alternatively known as a time motion (TM) scanner, time position (TP) scanner, motion (M-mode) scanner, echocardiograph, or ultrasonic cardiograph (UCG), this is an ultrasonic scanner which traces the movements of reflecting tissue interfaces with time. It is used primarily to study the action of the heart, particularly the valves, but is also used to study the movement of blood vessels and foetal heart.

The apparatus consists of an A-scanner with the hand-held transducer positioned over the heart. The A-scan signal is turned into a single-line B-scan (i.e. the intensity of the echoes is used to modulate the brightness of dots on a single line on the screen) and this line is swept slowly up or across the screen so that the movement of reflecting surfaces is seen. The image can be transferred to a permanent record via a fibre-optic recorder or Polaroid camera. The image is often presented alongside an ECG recording and/or phonocardiograph (PCG) to identify the timing of the events seen.

It comprises a high-voltage generator to activate the transducer, a receiving amplifier, a circuit to compensate for the absorption of sound with depth (time-gain compensation), a demodulator, and video amplifier to present the echoes as bright spots on the screen. A time-base is also required to generate the scan lines and move the line across the screen. Special circuits are often added to derive a varying voltage corresponding to the movement of a particular surface or heart valve leaflet.

Such devices are usually found in the cardiac department for the investigation of heart valve defects.

Magill attachment r=2

Alternatively called the Mapleson 'A' breathing circuit, this is the most commonly used of all breathing circuits for anaesthesia. It consists of a reservoir bag (not a rebreathing bag since exhaled gases should never reach it), a corrugated breathing tube, an expiratory valve, and a connection for a facepiece or endotracheal tube. Fresh gas is supplied at or slightly below the patient's minute volume through a feed at the bag end. When the patient exhales, most of the gases pass out through the expiratory valve, and so very little is rebreathed.

As a semi-closed breathing system it is satisfactory for spontaneous ventilation but the expiratory valve limits the pressure which can be applied during positive pressure ventilation. Increasing the blow-off pressure to prevent this is unsatisfactory.

Mammography system n=1 c=6 r=7

X-ray imaging of the breasts presents a special problem since they contain a range of soft tissues with little difference in their X-ray absorption. The solution is to provide soft X-rays with a photon energy of between 12 and 30 keV and it is usual to use a special X-ray set and tube. The tube usually has a molybdenum anode and a beryllium window and the X-ray cassette usually has a single fluorescent screen with a single emulsion film with very fine grain. Since the detail is important it is common to use vacuum cassettes to ensure intimate contact between the screens (if any) and the film.

Manley ventilator n=10, c=4 r=2

A range of lung ventilators has been designed for use during anaesthesia including minute volume dividers for open circuit anaesthesia (e.g. MP2 and Pulmovent) and high-pressure gas-driven types suitable for use with closed anaesthetic circuits (e.g. Manley Servovent). These provide assisted ventilation of the lungs during anaesthesia, taking a fresh gas feed from a continuous flow anaesthetic machine.

Mapleson breathing circuit r=2

Mapleson classified breathing circuits used in anaesthesia. The commonest type (the Mapleson A) is known also as the Magill attachment. Other types include variations in the position of the expiratory valve and fresh gas feed, the use of longer breathing tubes, or in the case of the Mapleson E there are no valves (T-piece circuit).

Marshall's indicator c=1 r=2

In paediatric anaesthesia a breathing circuit without valves (T-piece circuit) is often used because of its low resistance to spontaneous breathing. One problem with this is the absence of a basic breathing indicator as normally provided by the action of the expiratory valve. The Marshall's indicator is a foil flap mounted at the distal limb of the T-piece circuit, which can be seen moving in time with the breathing.

Masker

This is usually an integral part of a pure tone audiometer used for hearing tests in an audiology department. In audiometry, the performance of each ear is determined separately and the situation often arises (particularly in bone conduction tests) when the operator is not certain which ear is picking up the sound. Masking noise introduced into the non-test ear serves to make it temporarily deaf and so unable to detect the sounds directed to the test ear. When testing with pure tones (single frequencies) the masking noise is usually a narrow band of noise centred around the test frequency. In speech tests the masker may be wide band noise or 'speech shaped' noise.

The same problem arises when tuning fork tests are conducted by the ENT specialist. These crude tests have correspondingly crude maskers, for example rubbing a sheet of paper near the patient's non-test ear or using a device called a Barany box (see separate entry).

A tinnitus masker is a hearing aid-like device worn by patients suffering from tinnitus in order to cover up (mask) their own ear or head noises with an external masking noise.

Maskers are also used in the treatment of stammering (see Edinburgh masker). In this case the object is to prevent the subject from hearing his own voice.

Mass spectroscope/spectrograph n=2 c=5,6 r=6,9

A mass spectrometer is an apparatus which separates a stream of charged particles (ions) into a spectrum according to their mass-to-charge ratios and determines the relative abundance of each type of ion present. Medical mass spectrometers include a sample-inlet chamber, an ionization chamber, a dispersion chamber and an ion-detection (collection) system.

A thin sampling tube may connect the instrument to the site of recording (e.g. a lung ventilator). Gas is drawn into the sampling inlet chamber by a rotary pump reducing the pressure to 10–20 mmHg. A small amount of gas passes through a porous plug into an ionization chamber which is evacuated to approximately 1 part in 10 million of a mmHg. A stream of electrons travelling between a heated filament and anode bombard the gas entering the ionization chamber to produce ions. These ions are focused and accelerated in an electric field to the dispersion chamber where they are sorted into different molecular components. The sorting or dispersion techniques may include a magnetic field, quadripole electric field, or measurement of time of flight. The ion collector system produces an output for each type of ion involved. The inclusion of a circuit which sums all components in conjunction with the individual elements allows calculation of molar fractions.

In general the range is restricted to molecular weights of 4 (helium) to 44 (carbon dioxide). Extended ranges are possible to monitor hexafluoride (mass 146) and halothane (mass 196). Interference occurs between some molecules so that oxygen and carbon dioxide cannot be measured in the presence of either ether or nitrous oxide. Carbon monoxide interferes with nitrogen and nitrous oxide, although these can be measured with infrared instruments.

At present mass spectrometers are in use for research applications but have potential for patient monitoring in intensive care units. The rapid response time permits multiplexing of the sampling gas tubes so that gas mixtures from several patients, or several points in the same breathing circuit, can be recorded simultaneously. It is also possible to measure gases dissolved in tissues or blood by using a non-thrombogenic catheter with a semipermeable membrane covering its tip. Gases are drawn out of solution and through the membrane under the action of the inlet pump.

MAVIS (Movable Arterial and Venous Imaging System) n=1 c=6

MAVIS is a multichannel direction-resolving pulsed-wave ultrasonic doppler flow detector with imaging capability. The instrument can provide anterior–posterior, cross-sectional, and lateral views of blood vessels as well as the measurement of the velocity profiles across the vessel lumen. The major advantage over single-channel devices is the speed of measurement.

The system incorporates a position resolver, mechanically coupled to the ultrasound transducer. When the ultrasound beam is directed towards a blood vessel the presence of a flow signal is recorded as a spot on a storage monitor at a position corresponding to that of the probe. As the transducer is moved over the skin overlying the vessel, an image of its projection on the skin surface is generated on the screen.

MAVIS has 30 flow detection channels, each measuring the magnitude and direction of blood flow along the beam axis. The distance between the transducer and the first of the 30 detection points and the separation of the points are both variable. This allows superficial vessels to be imaged with a resolution of about 1 mm.

The beam angle is calculated using a microprocessor. Three cross-sectional scans about half a centimetre apart are required for this measurement. The distortion of the velocity profiles in the smaller vessels due to the finite size of the sampling volumes is also corrected by means of the microprocessor.

Such devices would be used in the investigation of arterial disease.

McKesson breathing circuits r=2

These are a set of connection arrangements for the anaesthetic circuit when using demand flow apparatus of the type used in dental anaesthesia and for some minor surgery.

McKesson expiratory valve c=1 r=2

Intended for nasal inhalers in dental anaesthesia, this is a spring-loaded disc valve on which the opening pressure can be adjusted on a calibrated clutch. This was useful when a degree of rebreathing against a spring loaded bag was required, but is not often used now.

McKesson inhaler c=1 r=2

A breathing circuit for use in dental anaesthesia and with demand flow apparatus. It consists of a nosepiece fitted with an expiratory valve, and also a mouthpiece to which the supply of gas is disrupted if it hangs down. It has a special connector to link the mouthpiece, the two tubes to the nosepiece, and the inlet.

Mechanical thumb ventilator n=1 c=4 r=2

For artificial ventilation in a T-piece circuit (valveless) used particularly for anaesthesia in infants, this device uses an electrically operated solenoid to block the free end of the breathing tube during inspiration so that the lungs are inflated by the fresh gas feed. The solenoid is released during expiration so that the patient can exhale by elastic recoil of the lungs. The control unit consists of timing devices and perhaps a pressure gauge. The Sheffield paediatric ventilator and the Amsterdam infant ventilator are machines of this type.

Medical compressed air r=2

Whether delivered in cylinders at the point of use or provided in a pipeline system, air for breathing must be carefully filtered to remove oil droplets and other debris.

A medical air supply may also be used for other purposes such as driving air-operated drills and saws, and for driving ventilators. Free-standing pumps are also available for generating clean air for breathing machines. Piped medical air is usually delivered at 4 or 7 bar (60 or 105 psi).

Memory oscilloscope n=60 c=4 r=3

To display a graph, or a signal which varies with time (e.g. ECG or arterial pressure) it is now usual to employ a short-persistence CRT in conjunction

167

with a simple computer memory. The memory is usually a 'first in first out' (FIFO) set of shift registers operating rather like a tape loop. The contents of the memory are read repeatedly on to the screen giving a frozen display, or if new information is being added to the memory this is added at one end of the line so the whole line appears to be moving slowly backwards or forwards. The older information is being discarded from the other end of the line.

Memory 'scopes have almost totally replaced long-persistence CRTs ('bouncing ball' or 'comet's tail' types) for ECG and blood pressure display.

The same principle can be used to form a whole image (as opposed to a single line) on the screen for ultrasonic B-scan display, and for images formed during isotope scanning. However, the memory requirements are much larger (e.g. 512×512 picture elements) and in the case of ultrasonic scanning the required speed of memory access is near to the practical limit. In these applications the memory is also used to convert the scanning method to a (TV) video format.

Mercury manometer n=300 c=1 r=2

Blood pressure measurement by sphygmomanometer is normally performed using a mercury manometer. This can consist of a U-tube half-filled with mercury, but more commonly it is a single tube, held vertical in use, which sits in a small reservoir of mercury. The reservoir is connected by a rubber tube to the source of air pressure to be measured. As pressure is applied mercury is forced up the column and the pressure can be read from a scale behind. The actual pressure is indicated by the difference in the level of the mercury in the column and the reservoir. Thus, the relative areas of the surfaces of the two sections of the device must be such that the reservoir level does not descend much due to the volume of mercury forced up the column during measurement.

This type of manometer is slow acting and cumbersome but has the advantage that it cannot give incorrect readings and, due to the high specific gravity of mercury (13.6), only a short tube is required to indicate the full range of possible blood pressures. Normally it provides for measurement up to 300 mmHg.

Mercury plethysmograph n=1 c=2 r=9

An estimate of changes in body or limb volume may be made using a strain gauge around the chest or limb. The usual transducer for this is a silicone-rubber tube containing a thin thread of mercury. As volume changes occur the strain gauge will exhibit changes in resistance which can be detected in a suitable bridge circuit. The best known application of this device is the venous occlusion plethysmograph in which pulsation in the limb may be detected, or more commonly the blood perfusion rate may be estimated by restricting the venous return from the limb for a short period (by a pressure cuff at say 50 mmHg) and recording the rate of rise of volume of the limb or limb segment. Similar information may be gained using inflated cuffs around the limb coupled to air flow or pressure transducers.

Such devices might be used by vascular or orthopaedic surgeons to assess the quality of blood perfusion in diseased limbs.

Metal fragment detector n=1 c=4

Small metal fragments can be extremely hard to find in a wound. A device exists which works in the same way as metal detectors used for finding pipes in walls and coins in the ground. The normal form of the instrument is a small suitcase unit with a long probe which can be placed very close to the wound, or a sterile latex sheath or finger from a surgical glove can be placed over the tip so that it may be allowed to touch the open wound.

The approach to a metal fragment is usually indicated by a change in pitch of a tone produced by the instrument. Such an instrument would be found in the casualty department.

Microelectrode r=9

In studying the electrophysiology of cells it is often necessary to measure the potential difference across the cell membrane. To do this the electrode must measure from within the cell. Very small electrodes can be made with tip sizes ranging from 0.05 to 10 μm. They may be formed from solid metal needles, metal contained within or on the surface of glass needles, or from a glass micropipette having the lumen filled with electrolytic solution. The electrode must be used with a special micromanipulator to enable the tip to be moved with precision through the cell wall.

Microtome n=3 c=4,5

This describes a range of instruments for cutting thin sections of tissue for examination under a microscope. Samples may be stiffened by embedding in paraffin wax or new plastic compounds, or by freezing. The instrument consists of a sample handler, a knife, and an inching mechanism to select the cut, thickness and angle required.

Microwave diathermy apparatus n=4 c=4 r=4,10

Heat treatment is used in the physiotherapy department to deal with pain, muscle spasm, stiffness and chronic inflammation. The heat may be applied by conduction through the skin, or diathermy may be used. One form of diathermy employs microwaves directed at the region to be treated from an antenna placed a short distance (10 or 20 cm) from the skin. The waves will pass a few centimetres into the body before they are completely absorbed, releasing heat into the tissue. The mechanism of operation is similar to that employed in microwave ovens. The usual frequency is 2450 MHz at which penetration may be up to 30 mm. The size of the area to be treated can be determined by the antenna design and the distance from the body.

These devices are normally used without monitoring the intensity levels or field patterns. Eye protection should be worn by patient and user.

Midliner $n=1$ $c=4$ $r=1$

This is a trade name for an ultrasonic A-scanner which automatically computes the position and displacement of the membranes (falx cerebri) separating the two lobes of the brain. It does not display the A-scan but identifies the large echoes representing the near and far side skull positions and examines the central area for echoes which could represent the falx cerebri. As the probe is manipulated on the skin above the ear the midliner presents numbers which represent the position of the midline echo in millimetres from the central position. The operator fills in a small chart with the results until there are sufficient to give a statistically correct indication of its position while ignoring the occasional incorrect result. The device is claimed to significantly reduce the number of incorrect diagnoses of shift of the midline.

Minute volume divider $n=10$ $c=3,4$ $r=2$

This is an open-circuit lung ventilator which derives its power from the pressure of gases delivered to it from a continuous-flow anaesthetic machine. The fresh gas feed must be at least equal to the minute volume requirement of the patient. A minute volume divider normally consists of an elastic or spring-loaded reservoir bag or bellows and a set of valves which allow the contents of the bellows to inflate the lungs at intervals. During the expiratory phase, while the bag is refilling, the patient's expired gases are exhausted to atmosphere.

The cycle time and the inspiratory to expiratory time (I:E ratio) are determined by a mechanism which may depend on time, volume, pressure or flow rate. A separate bellows may be provided to generate a negative pressure during the expiratory phase to draw gas out of the lungs. Examples of minute volume dividers are the Autovent, Minivent, Manley MP2 and Pulmovent, and the Philips AV1 adult/paediatric ventilator.

170

Modem

This is a modulator/demodulator for the transmission of computer information over telephone lines. It changes the signals into a form suitable for telephone lines. The most well-known type of instrument receives an ordinary telephone handset into two rubber cups which present acoustic information to the microphone, usually bleeping tones, and detect the tones received down the line and convert them into pulses suitable for the particular computer being used. The main limitation of this method is the slow rate at which information can be handled (usually 300 bits/s). To operate at higher speeds it is usual for the modem to be connected directly to the telephone line so that information may be transmitted as a series of electrical pulse codes, although tones are often used.

Monitored defibrillator n=10 c=4 r=3,4,6

Since defibrillators are intended to restart the heart, an electrocardiograph is normally required to confirm faulty action of the heart and to demonstrate return to normal action after the treatment has been applied. Thus, many modern defibrillators have a cardioscope (and/or cardiograph) built into them so that the diagnosis, the treatment, and the confirmation of success (or otherwise), can be made. These units are linked so that the cardioscope is not disabled by the defibrillator pulse. Also it is common for the ECG signal to be picked up through the defibrillator 'paddles' when they are applied to the chest.

A completely separate reason for linking a defibrillator and cardioscope is for synchronized defibrillation (sometimes called cardioversion).

On some units an ECG recorder (writer) may be included.

Monochromator r=9

This is a component of a spectrophotometer and may be a glass or quartz prism, or a diffraction grating. Its purpose is to divide a source of light or emission from a chemical sample into a spectrum of wavelengths from which one or more may be selected for passing to a photometer.

Motorized syringe n=50 c=2 r=4

This is an automatic device for slowly discharging the contents of a syringe through a cannula into a vein. It is normally a simple electromechanical device, often employing a stepping motor to drive a gearbox coupled to a worm drive which drives the plunger of a syringe. It is often called an infusion pump or syringe pump.

MR scanner n=1 c=8

Previously known as a nuclear magnetic resonance (NMR) scanner, the word 'nuclear' has been dropped to avoid confusion with devices producing harmful radiations. This can produce images of selected planes within the body which are similar in general appearance to CT scans, but the image relates to the state and content of water at each point within the scan plane.

The technique has the potential to identify other aspects of the chemical structure of tissues but at present medical imaging is limited to information derived from the spin resonance of the hydrogen nucleus. The hydrogen nucleus forms a small magnet which will absorb and emit radio-frequency energy at a resonant frequency depending on the strength of an applied magnetic field. By the application of a magnetic field gradient the resonant frequency will depend on position in the field. An extension of this principle allows the construction of 2- and 3-dimensional images.

The scanners currently available have solved the various construction problems (particularly those of the large magnets required) in various ways, but it will probably be some years before MR imaging facilities are generally available, partly because of the high capital and operating costs. A major advantage of an MR scanner is that there are no (known) harmful effects.

Multichannel analyser n=3 c=4 r=3

This could refer to any type of analyser (e.g. chemical analyser or frequency analyser) and the term is sometimes applied to devices used in nuclear medicine to collect the number of counts occurring at different pulse heights (different gamma-ray energies). In this latter case a graph or histogram may be plotted showing count rates resulting from different isotopes. Typically there may be 256 channels although there may be as many as 4096.

They are often small computers which can also operate on the results to subtract the counts due to the background radiation leaving only that due to radioactive isotopes in the body. They are often used on whole body scanners.

In clinical chemistry this term may refer to a large analyser (discrete or continuous flow) for performing several tests on each sample.

Multiformat camera n=1 c=3,4

Ultrasonic scans are often presented as small black and white prints taken from the screen of a small video monitor, using an instant camera. An alternative storage method which has become popular is to arrange six such pictures on a single sheet of X-ray film, using a multiformat camera.

In its simplest form, this is a special back for the camera, which holds the large film in a cassette which has a mechanism to allow the film to be moved into six positions. After taking the first picture, the operator moves the film to the next position, and so on.

There are a number of multiformat cameras in which the relocation process is automatic, and after loading the film cassette into the camera, the six pictures can be taken without operator intervention. After the pictures have been taken, the film is processed in the same way as X-ray film.

It must be remembered that the film produces a negative image. This is normally dealt with by inverting the video signal applied to the video monitor.

Myophone

This term has been used to describe an instrument which uses surface electrodes to pick up small signals due to muscle activity and translate them into a sound signal whose intensity is related to the level of activity in the muscle under the electrode. This may be used as an indicator of arousal in response to auditory stimulus to assist the therapist to train the patient. In some ways this is similar to the relaxometer.

N

Nasal anemometer n=3 c=3

This measures the rate of air flow in litres/minute in the nose. The patient dons a rubber mask fitted with an electrically heated thermistor bead. The flow of air down the nose cools the bead and an electronic conditioning amplifier converts this into air flow rate. This is useful for objective assessment before, during, and after treatment of the hypernasal patient and may be used in the speech therapy department. Similar devices also exist for use in the intensive care department to monitor the flow through the nose or simply to monitor or record breathing patterns.

Nebulizer n=400 c=2 r=2

This is a device for increasing the humidity of air, oxygen, or anaesthetic gases to be breathed by a patient. Increase in humidity is achieved in a nebulizer by creating many tiny droplets of water in the airstream to the patient. The patient receives the extra moisture whether or not evaporation actually occurs. Methods of nebulizing water into the airway include bubbling the gas through water, a jet of gas or air may be used to entrain water, a fine jet of water may be made to impinge on a surface or baffles in an airway, or high-intensity ultrasound may be employed to project droplets from the surface of water. Nebulizers of various types are also used for the dispersal of antiseptics during the sterilization of breathing machines. A fan may be used to assist the flow of air.

The drop size is most important since large drops may waterlog the airways without reaching the alveoli, and very small drops may humidify the alveoli without effect on the airways.

Nephelometer n=3 c=3 n=5

Information about a colloidal suspension can be obtained from the amount of light scattered. The sample is illuminated from one side and the amount of light scattered sideways is detected. A clear solution should not scatter any of the light. Such devices are occasionally used in the clinical chemistry department.

Nephroscope n=2 c=3,4

This is usually a rigid endoscope with rod lenses for viewing directly inside the kidney through a dorsal puncture. In common with other endoscopes it has channels for irrigation, and instruments such as grasping and crushing tools, or for ultrasonic and electrohydraulic probes for stone breaking.

Nerve stimulator n=12 c=2,3 r=3

Electrical stimulation of nerves is performed for a variety of reasons. Anaesthetists use battery-operated stimulators which present short-duration high-voltage pulses to the skin to determine whether the effect of muscle relaxants used during surgery is sufficient to suppress all function of the voluntary muscles. Stimulators which may affect the nerves are also used for the relief of pain. These use lower voltages and do not usually cause muscle contraction. In the physiotherapy department electrical stimulators are widely used in order to exercise muscles: whether they act directly on the muscle or via nerves is probably not important.

Nerve stimulators are also used in a range of diagnostic procedures. In the neurology department nerves are stimulated via skin electrodes or via needle electrodes which may be placed right into the nerve trunk. A typical reason for stimulating the muscle in this way is to establish the conduction velocity of the longer nerves, which is diagnostic of certain diseases, and a low velocity may suggest that the nerve is trapped at some point. Most conduction velocity tests are performed on the efferent (motor) nerves but the same stimulation can be applied to the afferent (sensory) nerves, but this is less often done since the response further along the nerve is more difficult to detect.

A nerve stimulator consists of a pulse generator of variable rate, a pulse length controller, an amplifier, and an isolating circuit. Cardiac pacemakers may also be considered to be nerve stimulators.

Neutral electrode

This term is synonymous with 'indifferent electrode' as used in monopolar surgical diathermy. It is a metal or metallized plastic flexible plate of relatively large area (e.g. 10 cm × 10 cm) for connection to the body of the patient to provide a return path for the high-frequency current used in surgical diathermy, but with such a low current density at the skin that the physical effects which might cause burns are avoided.

Nitrogen analyser n=1 c=4 r=9

This is usually an emission spectroscope which is used in medical work to calculate the molar fraction of nitrogen in a gas mixture. It is used in some lung function tests.

A tiny quantity of the gas mixture to be sampled is drawn through a needle valve by a high vacuum pump to provide pressures of 1 to 4 mmHg and this gas mixture is ionized between two electrodes in an ionization chamber. The gases emit light which is detected by a phototube after passing through an optical filter to remove wavelengths outside the range of 310–480 nm. An amplifier and linearizing circuit are connected to the phototube to produce a figure for nitrogen concentration. Nitrogen concentration from 0 to 80% can be measured with considerable accuracy with response time of the order of 40 ms. Oxygen and carbon dioxide do not interfere with the accuracy, but helium and argon can produce errors.

Nuclear magnetic resonance (NMR) scanner n=1 c=8

The term nuclear magnetic resonance (NMR) scanner has now been dropped in favour of magnetic resonance (MR), to avoid confusion with devices producing harmful radiations. See MR Scanner.

Nystagmograph n=2 c=3,4

More often called an electronystagmograph (see separate entry), nystagmograph equipment is used for the objective measurement of eye movement (nystagmus), usually for the investigation of vertigo and balance impairment.

O

Octave band analyser n=1 c=4 r=8

Most sound level meters include an amplifying circuit designed to approximate to the frequency response of the human ear and so make the readings more relevant in terms of perceived loudness. If a more objective analysis of sound is required it is useful to make readings of sound pressure in restricted frequency bands or ranges and so obtain an idea of the spectrum of the sounds present.

An octave band analyser is a series of electronic filters having a pass-band of one octave each. The device is usually an add-on accessory for a sound level meter.

Octoson r=1

This is a trade name for an unusual type of ultrasonic B-scanner which is fully automatic. The patient lies on a special table which has a large membrane at its centre smeared with ultrasonic coupling jelly on to which the patient presses the area to be scanned. For an abdominal scan the patient is face down with the abdominal skin in contact with the membrane. In the case of infants they are laid on this membrane. Beneath the membrane is a large water tank partially supporting the membrane and in the bottom of this is an array of ultrasonic transducers which are large, long focal length, dish transducers. A compound scan is performed by the rocking of these transducers while the image is being formed.

Very high-quality images can be produced by this method.

Oesophageal pacemaker n=1 c=2,3

Defibrillation is ineffective in treating some heart attack victims. External pacing can help, but in emergency situations valuable time is lost in inserting a cardiac catheter. Using an oesophageal pacemaker the pacing catheter is inserted transorally or transnasally in 30 seconds or so.

Approximately 30 V output is required for the pacer to achieve cardiac pacing.

177

Oesophageal stethoscope r=4

After the induction of anaesthesia, heart and lung sounds may be monitored very successfully using a balloon-tipped tube inserted into the oesophagus via the mouth. This oesophageal stethoscope may also be used as a channel for other sensors such as thermistors or electrodes.

Oil heating bath r=9

These are used in continuous-flow automated chemical analysers to accelerate colour reactions. See Auto analysers.

Open circuit r=2

Although this has an electrical meaning, it also refers to a type of breathing circuit used in anaesthesia in which the mask does not fit the face and there is free access of air to the breathing circuit. It may also refer to anaesthetic or ventilator circuits in which the gases exhaled are passed directly out of the breathing circuit with no intentional rebreathing.

Open drop mask c=1 r=2

A face mask for anaesthesia on to which ether, chloroform or other volatile agent is administered as drops on to a lint.

Ophthalmodynamometer

Information about the systolic and diastolic pressure occurring in the ophthalmic artery, and also about the pulse wave velocity of the internal carotid artery can be determined by simultaneously recording pressure within the eye and pressure within the brachial artery. Equipment exists to measure these two parameters simultaneously; the pulsations within the eye are detected using an applanation tonometer. Such apparatus is not often found.

Ophthalmometer

This is designed to accurately measure the curvature of the anterior surface of the cornea, which is the chief refracting surface of the human eye. It can thus deliver a primary index of the patient's astigmatism. Measurements are made either in millimetres radius of curvature or in dioptres. It is an optical device which reflects an image off the surface of the cornea to an observing screen.

Ophthalmoscope n=50 c=1

This instrument is a hand-held device containing a battery in the handle, a bulb for illuminating the inside of the eye, and a set of lenses set in a disc which can be rotated to select different strengths. The device is held in front of the patient's eye and the operator looks through one of the small lenses into the eye to view the appearance of the cornea, the lens, the aqueous and vitreous humour, and the surface of the retina. The blood vessels in the retina can be clearly seen and there are particular appearances for diseases such as diabetes mellitus, hypertension, and other conditions. Some hereditary disorders of the retina also produce characteristic appearances.

Optokinetic drum n=2 c=2

A vertical cylinder about 20 cm in diameter marked with black and white vertical stripes is rotated by motor or by hand while the patient follows the stripes with his eyes. Brain stem lesions which impair the ability to follow moving objects can be detected. Eye movements may be monitored visually or by electronystagmograph apparatus. These may be found in orthoptic and audiology departments.

Orthosis

This is a general term for an external mechanical device intended to replace or supplement the mechanical functions of joints or muscles. An example of an orthosis is a set of leg calipers.

Orthovoltage X-ray set n=1 c=6,7

A therapy X-ray set which uses a conventional X-ray tube to emit X-rays in the range of 100–500 keV. These sets will be used with either open or closed-ended applicators. The focal point to skin distance (FSD) is fixed by the length of the applicator. Metal filters are frequently used in the X-ray beam to 'harden' the beam by reducing the emission of the lower energy X-rays. They are used to treat both superficial and other lesions but not those which are deep seated. Orthovoltage X-ray sets are found in radiotherapy departments.

Oscillating saw n=6 c=4

Hand saws looking very like carpenters' saws are sometimes used for working on large bones. However, there are power saws available which fall into electric and pneumatic types. The electric type may have a blade which vibrates and is used for splitting the sternum at the start of chest surgery. The advantage of having a vibrating rather than a rotating blade is that, if the vibrations are small, cutting will only occur in hard materials (e.g. bone), but will not occur in soft materials. Compressed air powered drills are more common, particularly for orthopaedic surgery. They often come as a kit consisting of an air-operated motor and foot-operated speed control, and a set of fittings for sawing, drilling, screwing and pinning. They are intended to work from nitrogen or air at 7 bar pressure which may be provided by pipeline or from cylinders.

Since the surgeon normally holds the motor during the sawing operation the whole device must be sterilizable. Pneumatic types are more amenable to total sterilization.

Electric oscillating saws are also used for cutting plaster casts.

Oscillometer n=30 c=1 r=2

This is a device for intermittent indirect blood pressure measurement which uses a double cuff on the upper arm, and is commonly used by anaesthetists. It is also called an oscillotonometer, and a description of its operation is given under that heading.

Oscilloscope n=4 c=3,4 r=3

This is an instrument containing a cathode ray tube (CRT) intended for viewing signals that vary with time. There are different types of oscilloscope but the most common format is a short-persistence CRT with amplifiers driving the vertical (Y) deflection plates and a time base driving the horizontal (X) deflection plates. The amplifiers usually have variable gain and sometimes filtering circuits; the time base allows the horizontal sweep of the spot to be made at different speeds. Other variations are to have a storage CRT or electronic storage circuits, X and Y drive amplifiers (i.e. no time base), differential amplifiers, special time base triggering circuits, etc.

General-purpose oscilloscopes are only found in electronics research or servicing laboratories; however, the common cardioscope is in fact an oscilloscope with a time-base, a differential amplifier with filters, and a long-persistence CRT or memory circuit. However, one does not usually think of them as oscilloscopes.

Because of their versatility, it is often convenient to use an industrial oscilloscope as the display for a medical measuring instrument. In these circumstances care should be taken to ensure there is no breach of the recommendations relating to the use of electrical equipment in the patient environment.

180

Oscillotonometer n=30 c=1 r=2,6

Intermittent indirect blood pressure measurement can be conducted in the operating theatre by use of an oscillotonometer (sometimes called an oscillometer). This has two inflatable cuffs on the upper arm which connect via rubber tubes to a control unit, which looks like a large size aneroid pressure gauge but in fact contains two aneroid capsules which can be connected up to provide a differential pressure between the cuffs, or a single pressure (when the cuffs are connected together).

In operation, the cuffs are inflated together to above the systolic pressure using the usual bulb-type pump. The pressure is gradually released, and from time to time a switch is operated to change the internal connection between the two cuffs so that the lower cuff senses the pulsations due to arterial wall movement. These pulsations are at a maximum when the upper cuff is at the systolic pressure. They fall gradually from this point and practically disappear at the diastolic pressure. The aneroid capsules are cleverly linked inside so that the gauge shows the pressure being applied to the upper cuff with the pulsations from the lower cuff superimposed.

Other equipment exists which utilizes double-cuff methods and electronic processing of the pressure and pulse signals. An example is described under Haemotonometer.

Osmometer n=3 c=4 r=6

Solutes or ions in water cause a lowering of the freezing point. The magnitude of the freezing point depression depends on the number of particles per kilogram of water and this number is expressed in Osmols where one Osmol is Avogadro's number of particles per kilogram. Blood or urine osmolality measurements may be required for patients in intensive care. An osmometer measures osmolality by detecting the 'freezing point depression'. At one Osmol, the freezing point is 1.858°C below normal.

Freezing point is found by detecting the temperature at which a small quantity of the fluid (e.g. 3 ml) freezes in a small cuvette. A small stirrer or vibrator and a thermistor probe are immersed in the fluid and the cuvette is lowered into a freezing bath or Peltier cooling device. The stirrer is arrested by the freezing of the solution and this triggers the measurement of temperature. True freezing point is measured just after the first freezing and this is slightly higher than the lowest temperature reached. The instrument displays osmolality directly. It may also be called an osmolality, or osmolarity meter.

Otoacoustic emission processor/audiometer n=1 c=5

It has been discovered that the cochlea can emit sound as well as detect it.

Further, it will produce a small sound in response to a sound stimulus, but this response is diminished or absent in the case of hearing loss of cochlear origin.

This discovery is the basis of a new technique and apparatus for assessing cochlea hearing loss which provides a click stimulus to the outer ear and then detects and analyses the acoustic response of the cochlea. This uses frequency analysis to compare the response with the stimulus, and it is claimed that the extent and frequency dependence of hearing loss can be predicted from a comparison of the spectral content of the stimulus and response. For each person there is a characteristic 'cochlea echo' which can be recorded and used as a reference in future testing.

This is a new device which should be extremely useful in the assessment of noise-induced hearing loss, and for objective audiometry in a wide range of situations. The main advantage over alternative techniques (for instance electrocochleography) is that it is non-invasive.

Otoscope n=50 c=1

Also known as an auriscope, the otoscope is a hand-held battery-powered light source and lens system for looking into the outer ear. Most have a detachable tip (speculum) which comes in a range of sizes. The bulb is usually energized via a rheostat (variable resistance) in order to control its brightness although this facility is normally used only in ophthalmic testing when the lens and speculum are detached and replaced by an ophthalmoscope attachment. Most otoscopes are monocular devices although binocular versions are available.

Overhead baby warmer n=5 c=4

As a substitute for an enclosed canopy incubator to keep small babies warm during observation and treatment an overhead baby warmer may be used. This consists of a cot with a heating device mounted on an arm overhead. The overhead heater may use incandescent filament (infrared) lamps with a special glass filter to reduce visible and ultraviolet radiation or it may deliver non-visible light from overwound or enclosed elements of the types used in domestic electrical heaters.

Oximeter n=3 c=3 r=2,9

This is usually a device which can distinguish between oxyhaemoglobin and reduced haemoglobin by measuring and comparing the absorption of red and infrared light. Bench models exist which take blood in a cuvette, but the technique can also be applied *in vivo*. *In vivo* models usually clip on to the ear and shine light through the ear-lobe (the heat from the lamp also acts to increase the blood circulation in the ear). On the other side of the ear-lobe are filters and photocells.

The *in vivo* devices have not found wide acceptance because there are errors due to the quality of the blood being sampled (i.e. it is not arterial blood), small falls in the oxygen content of the blood cannot be detected, and biological variations in the total haemoglobin level render a single measurement inaccurate.

The technique is much more accurate if blood samples can be taken, especially if blood can be haemolysed (red cells ruptured). This can be done completely outside the body but in the cardiac catheterization laboratory blood samples may be drawn down the catheter for on-line analysis. This is particularly useful in identifying leaks between the chambers of the heart that may occur in some septal defects. The oxyhaemoglobin content of the right heart would be raised if blood from the left heart were able to leak through. In some models the light absorption/reflection characteristics of the blood are detected remotely using fibre-optic coupling from the external measuring device to the blood inside the body.

Use of a fibre-optic oximeter can improve speed of response of cardiac output estimation and provide intensive care monitoring of blood oxygen saturation.

Oxygen analyser n=20 c=2,3,4 r=6

There are a number of situations in anaesthesia and intensive care where it is important to measure the oxygen concentration. In addition, oxygen analysers are important tools in the checking of oxygen therapy and anaesthetic apparatus for correct performance.

There are three main types found in hospitals:

1. Paramagnetic analysers. Oxygen is unique among gases in that it is paramagnetic (moves towards stronger magnetic fields) whereas most other gases are diamagnetic (move away). In the paramagnetic analyser (see separate entry) a small glass bulb of nitrogen experiences a force acting towards a weaker part of a magnetic field when the gas surrounding it is diamagnetic. Such devices can be made fast acting, highly accurate and durable.
2. Fuel cell analysers. Oxygen diffuses through a permeable membrane (usually PTFE – Teflon) at a rate dependent on the concentration and this oxygen feeds a chemical reaction leading to the production of a small electrical current. These take 30 seconds or so to reach equilibrium and the cells normally only last for a few months.
3. Polarographic electrodes. This uses the Clark electrode in which oxygen

diffuses through a PTFE membrane into a solution containing a platinum cathode and a silver–silver chloride reference electrode. Oxygen dissociates in the presence of water and a small potential between the electrodes (usually 0.6 V). This produces a very small current between the electrodes which is amplified and displayed. The electrodes do not last indefinitely.

Oxygen bypass (flush) control r=2

This is a manually operated valve on a continuous flow anaesthetic machine which causes oxygen to bypass the the rotameters and back bar for flushing the breathing circuit, and for use in emergencies.

Oxygen concentrator n=3 c=4

An alternative to using piped or bottled oxygen to enrich the air supply to patients with lung disorders is to use an oxygen concentrator. This employs a 'molecular sieve' which is a mechanical filter which allows smaller molecules through more easily. Air is drawn through the sieve and the initial gas mixture delivered has an enhanced oxygen level. This mixture is retained, the system purged, and the process repeated. The retained gases are fed through the sieve repeatedly to progressively enhance the oxygen concentration. Usually two sieves are in use which work alternately. Portable units are available which are suitable for use by the patient at home, thus removing the need for bottled gas deliveries.

Oxygen failure warning device r=2

If the oxygen supply fails during anaesthesia or artificial ventilation the consequences may be disastrous, particularly if the nitrous oxide supply to the patient continues. Various types of oxygen failure warning device exist for inclusion on anaesthetic apparatus and breathing machines, and in oxygen pipelines. The simplest types include a Bosun's whistle in which a small bellows is held in the inflated state by the pressure of the oxygen supply. When the supply fails this bellows collapses, blowing a whistle. One type (the Bosun) also has a battery operated light, but most modern types incorporate a device for the automatic disconnection of other gases (or at least the nitrous oxide) should the oxygen fail or run out. Examples of oxygen failure warning devices include the Gardiner safety interlock, and types made by BOC, Vickers, Penlon, and EGC.

Unfortunately the introduction of these devices has been marred by occasional failure.

Oxygen hood r=4

In cases of respiratory distress syndrome in newborns a small plastic box which opens on one side is placed over the baby's head and a humidified oxygen-enriched atmosphere supplied. This is more efficient than using a chamber containing the whole infant.

Oxygenator r=4

During heart surgery the function of the heart and lungs must be undertaken outside the body, in a heart–lung machine. Lung function is emulated in an oxygenator which must supply fresh oxygen to the blood and remove carbon dioxide. There are two main types of oxygenator: those involving direct contact between the gas and the blood and those in which the gases are required to diffuse through membranes.

The features which are sought in an oxygenator are efficient transfer, minimum blood trauma, safety and reliability, low cost and small blood priming volume.

Direct contact oxygenators are usually bubble oxygenators in which the blood passes up a column, and bubbles of oxygen rise through it. As the oxygen is taken up by the blood, carbon dioxide is released and this is vented at the top. There are many designs of columns to ensure that there is good mixing and contact between the gas and the blood. This may be a series of tubes or some kind of baffles to promote mixing. At the top of the column the blood forms a foam which must be coalesced into a reservoir. It then passes through a filter and a bubble trap.

Membrane oxygenators use a thin semipermeable membrane to separate the blood and gas phases. There is some blood trauma due to the denaturing of plasma proteins and damaging of blood cells which limits perfusion to a few hours, but these problems may be minimized by better materials for the membrane. Such oxygenators also have application in organ preservation for transplantation.

The membranes may be flat plates or closely spaced tubes. However, current membrane materials cannot be scaled to provide transfer efficiencies equivalent to the natural lung, and extra design features must be included to cause turbulence in the blood film.

P

Pacemaker n=50 c=3 r=3,6

Heart block is the incorrect generation or transmission of the natural pacing pulses arising from the sinoatrial node. The problem may be congenital or may result from cardiac surgery or heart disease. In such cases a common treatment is to use an electronic pacemaker to present pacing pulses to the atrium or ventricles, depending upon the site of the disease or malfunction.

Pacemakers may be external devices connected to the heart via long catheters passed through a vein or even by electrodes placed in the oesophagus, but more commonly they are implanted devices operating from internal batteries or via an inductive link to an external power source. There are two basic types of device, the fixed rate pacemakers, and those which provide pacing pulses only when required. These latter types are called non-competitive or demand pacemakers because they pulse only when intrinsic activity fails.

There are many variations on these themes, summarised by the following abbreviations:

AAT   Triggered by atrial depolarization giving reinforcing stimulus to the atrium.
VOO   Asynchronous ventricular pacemaker.
VVI   Demand pacemaker inhibited by ventricular depolarization.
VVT   Triggered by ventricular depolarization giving a reinforcing stimulus to the ventricles.
DVI   Stimulating both chambers sequentially but inhibited by ventricular polarization.

The pacing may be unipolar or bipolar. In the bipolar case the two electrodes are mounted on the tip of the pacing catheter. In unipolar stimulation a single electrode is in the heart muscle while the other is elsewhere, usually mounted on the pacemaker itself.

The power source for implanted pacemakers may be batteries which require replacement every few years, of which the lithium–iodine cells are now the most attractive (up to ten years' life). Alternatively, a nuclear-powered pacemaker may last longer than this, using plutonium-238 or promethium-147. The life of plutonium cells may exceed ten years.

Pacing leads and electrodes must produce minimal electrochemical reaction and also withstand flexing and corrosion. They are normally helical coils of platinum–irridium alloys encapsulated in silicon rubber. The electrodes are often helical coils which screw into the heart muscle, thus simplifying the implantation procedures. If the pacemaker must be changed for any reason it is common for the same electrodes to be used.

The term pacemaker is sometimes used incorrectly to describe other forms of electrical stimulator such as those used for bladder or urethral muscle stimulation.

Pacemaker analyser n=1 c=4 r=3

Patients with implanted pacemakers are asked to attend a clinic at regular intervals to evaluate the performance of their pacemaker. The procedure may involve ECG and X-ray tests. The electrocardiograms are to establish that pacing currents flow from the correct site in the heart to the second electrode (usually on the pacemaker), or the pacemaker may include circuits to transmit (usually by an inductive link) diagnostic information about its own performance. In this last case a special analyser may be supplied by the makers of the pacemaker to collect and interpret this information.

Such devices would be used in the cardiology department.

Panendoscope n=5 c=3 r=4

This is an endoscope providing a view directly along the axis of the telescope. This term is little used now since most recently introduced flexible endoscopes also use an end view. The term has been used to describe the urethroscope as distinct from a cystoscope, which normally views to the side.

Paramagnetic oxygen analyser n=5 c=4 r=6

Oxygen is unique among gases in that it is strongly paramagnetic. Thus it will move towards a stronger part of a magnetic field, whereas other gases are diamagnetic and move away. The device consists of a small glass dumbell with the bulbs filled with nitrogen (diamagnetic). These are placed between magnetic poles shaped to provide a gradient of magnetic field so that they tend to move in the direction of decreasing field strength. The dumbell is suspended at its centre on a torsion wire such that rotation occurs in proportion to the difference in magnetic properties between the nitrogen in the bulbs and the surrounding gas. The test gas is fed into the space between the magnetic poles such that the rotating force depends on the concentration of oxygen in the test gas.

A direct reading instrument can be constructed by fitting a small reflecting mirror on the dumbell, but more accurate and linear types employ electrostatic or magnetic feedback such that the rotating force is measured with only minimal movement. Such devices provide accurate, fast acting and robust oxygen analysers suitable for measuring oxygen in a wide range of gas mixtures.

Pasteurizer n=5 c=2 r=2

Sterilization of instruments which are damaged by high-temperature sterilization (e.g. by autoclaving) can be effected by heating in water to 70–75°C for a minimum of 20 minutes. This procedure kills most infective agents but is only really suitable for items where total sterility is not required. Repeated pasteurization may damage some items or reduce their anti-static properties. A pasteurizer usually takes the form of a small heated water bath.

Patient circuit r=2,10

Where the patient is included in an active, or measurement circuit, that part of circuit which shares current, energy, or gas flow with the patient is called the patient circuit. For electric circuits the topic is dealt with in BS 5724/IEC 601.1. Often the breathing circuit of anaesthetic apparatus is referred to as the patient circuit.

Pattern generator n=2 c=4

In the diagnosis of disorders of the visual system and in the investigation of some neural diseases which may also affect vision, it is common to measure the visual evoked potential (VEP), sometimes called the visual evoked response (VER). In this test a flash or pattern change stimulus is provided and the response is detected from electrodes over the visual cortex. The result is an electrical potential with characteristic waves demonstrating the passage of the signal through various stages of neural transmission and processing. The response is affected by background illumination, the intensity change occurring during the stimulus, and the change in the geometric pattern of the stimulating image. The effect of the intensity change can be eliminated by the use of a pattern reversal stimulator which changes from one image to the next without change in intensity.

The commonest form of this pattern stimulus is a checkerboard of black and white squares which alternates the black and white areas so that there is no change in average light level.

There are two main types of pattern generator. The first employs one or two slide projectors illuminating a screen with the alternate patterns by back projection. The second type uses a television type of cathode ray tube with a computer generator providing the patterns. A timing pulse is provided from the stimulator to the recording apparatus to start the measurement system at the time of reversal.

Such apparatus is used in the ophthalmology department or in the neurophysiology department.

Peak flowmeter n=10 c=2 r=2,3,6

This normally refers to a device for measuring the maximum expiratory flow rate as an aid to assessing lung function. It may be a dedicated device such as the Wright peak flowmeter, or the peak flow may be gleaned from a more general test instrument such as the Vitalograph or a recording spirometer.

In the case of the Wright peak flowmeter the peak expiratory flow rate (PEFR) can be measured in the ward or clinic by a simple hand-held instrument into which the patient blows. The flow of air is directed against a movable vane restrained by a spiral spring and as the vane moves further round the dial it uncovers more escape holes. There is a ratchet to hold the vane in the maximum position reached. Typical PEFR for an adult male is 7 l/s.

PEEP valve r=2

During the expiratory phase of intermittent positive pressure lung ventilation the small airways and the alveoli may close completely due to the low or negative pressure applied. This can be prevented by ensuring that there is a small positive pressure being applied at the end of expiration (PEEP). Some lung ventilators can provide PEEP by a restriction of the outflow of gases or by a special valve to allow expiration only above a specific pressure.

Penetrameter n=1 c=3,4

It is possible to estimate the kilovoltage applied to an X-ray tube without making a direct electrical connection to the X-ray set. The penetrameter is a test cassette in which an X-ray film is exposed with a pattern caused by the X-rays being attenuated by passing through layers of copper sheeting of different thickness.

The relationship between X-ray attenuation in copper and kilovoltage is well documented, and thus it is possible to calculate kilovoltage from densitometer readings of the exposure patterns using a table of values provided with the penetrameter.

The construction of the penetrameter is normally in seven layers:

1. The top cover
2. A copper sheet

3. A plastic sheet with alternate rows of copper discs set into it, and matching holes.
4. The intensifying screen
5. An optical attenuator
6. The X-ray film
7. The bottom cover.

In use it would be normal to expose the cassette several times at different kilovoltage settings, but masking different areas on the cassette with lead sheets. It would also be usual to expose a number of films in this way but at different mAs settings.

There are variations on this theme including the Wisconsin test cassette, and the Ardran-Crooks cassette.

Perimeter

This is for testing the field of vision. The subject places his chin on a rest and the eye to be tested is focused on a white disc in the centre of the apparatus. A second fixation target is slowly moved in from the periphery of vision and the subject indicates when he first sees it. By moving the second object in from various directions it is possible to map the field of vision. Various refinements on the basic instruments are available including automatic mapping, and circuits to detect if the eye wanders from the main fixation target. The visual field is drawn as a set of isopters for different target size, intensity, or colour.

Peripheral nerve stimulator n=10 c=2,3 r=3

This is an electrical device, usually battery operated, often used by anaesthetists to test for the effect of muscle relaxants during surgery. In its simplest form two ball electrodes protruding from the hand-held stimulator unit are pressed on to the skin over a nerve at the elbow or wrist. The electrical pulses are short (e.g. 100 μs) and of high voltage (up to 200 V) so that the nerve is stimulated even when it is at some distance from the skin. There will be a 'twitch' response of the muscles served by the nerve unless a blocking agent is in use.

Similar electrical stimulators are also required during tests of nerve conduction velocity, where the response to a stimulus is detected at two points along a nerve, and the difference in the response time used to calculate velocity. These stimulators are usually mains operated and can be triggered remotely.

Lower levels of stimulation are used for the relief of pain, using transcutaneous electrical neural stimulation (TENS).

Peristaltic pump n=50 c=3

The pumping of blood and other fluids which must not be contaminated is often performed using a peristaltic pump. A roller or vane squeezes a flexible tube against a shoe so forcing the fluid forward from the closed point of tube. The rollers or vanes may be on the outside of a rotating wheel, with sufficient (two or more) rollers/vanes to ensure that there is always at least one closed point in the tube, thus preventing back-flow. Roller pumps are commonly used in haemodialysis and in the heart/lung pump.

A very common type of pump for intravenous fluids also produces a peristaltic flow. The plastic tube leading from the bag or bottle on the drip stand to the intravenous needle (i.e. the 'giving set' or 'drip-set') passes through a special gate in which it is occluded between a row of 'fingers' which are moved by a cam mechanism to squeeze the closed point forward.

Peritoneal dialysis clamp

Kidney function may be partially replaced by peritoneal dialysis, which involves infusing a special solution (dialysate) into the potential space between the two membranes of the peritoneum (which surrounds most of the abdominal organs). The dialysate remains in the abdomen for a time (e.g. 1 hour) and is then drawn off, and new dialysate infused. It often employs an automatic timing device which clamps the outlet tube while fluid is fed in from a bag or bottle and clamps the inlet line while fluid is drawn off.

The device consists of a set of electrical or electronic timers and motorized gate valves which clamp the tubes at the correct times.

Peritoneal dialysis machine n=3 c=4 r=3,4

Where the function of the kidneys is impaired or absent some replacement of the lost function can be achieved by a process of dialysis, in which small molecular weight toxins (e.g. urea) are removed from the body by diffusion through a semipermeable membrane into a special dialysing fluid.

In haemodialysis, blood is removed from the body and passed over a dialysing membrane through which the toxins diffuse. In peritoneal dialysis, the dialysing fluid is passed through a surgically inserted tube, into a space between the two membranes of the peritoneum. The peritoneal membrane envelops most of the organs in the abdomen.

A peritoneal dialysis machine controls the passage of the dialysing fluid into the peritoneal cavity where the diffusion exchange takes place. It may also employ a weighing transducer to monitor the quantity of fluid infused. Some machines prepare the dialysing solution from a sterile concentrate, and water produced in a reverse osmosis column. After a period of time the fluid is withdrawn and a new solution infused. The machine itself is a set of valves, pumps and timers which control this process. Such devices are used in intensive care to remove natural toxins or drugs, and are also used in cases of renal failure.

Peritoneal dialysis is now widely used without automatic equipment, using a simple collapsible bag which the patient operates himself at home. This technique is called continuous ambulatory peritoneal dialysis (CAPD), and apart from the lessened restriction on the patient's lifestyle, it also reduces the risk of infection due to repeated connections of apparatus. Peritoneal dialysis, since it takes place inside the body, requires a much higher quality of dialysing fluid.

Perometer n=3 c=4 r=2

This is a blood loss meter for use after surgery to estimate the quantity of blood lost into swabs and drapes. It consists of a small washing machine in which the cloths are washed in a haemolytic solution, and a device for estimating the volume of blood in the wash. This may work on the colorimetric principle to measure the haemoglobin content, or it may measure the electrical impedance. The method is time consuming and so is not often used, and in any case its accuracy is limited since it cannot record the blood lost into the suction apparatus, on to the floor, or effectively lost as clots near the wound or injury.

pH meter n=5 c=3 r=9

The pH (hydrogen ion concentration or acidity) of samples of body fluids, including blood, may be measured as part of the chemical analysis of such samples. The pH meter has two electrodes, one for reference and one for measurement. The measurement electrode employs a membrane of special glass containing a solution of known pH. The approach of a hydrogen ion to the outside of the membrane causes a positive charge to pass into the ionic solution inside the electrode. The voltage developed across the electrode changes by approximately 60 mV/pH unit. Since the whole range of physiological pH values is only 0.6 pH units, the meter must be capable of accurately measuring changes of 0.1 mV. The reference electrode is usually a calomel cell in a potassium chloride salt bridge connecting with a porous plug at the tip of the electrode.

The voltage produced by a pH electrode varies with the temperature of the specimen, and so it is usual to maintain the test solution at 37°C, although the meter may also have a temperature correction control. The meter is normally calibrated by the use of two solutions of known pH. The internal impedance of the pH electrode is very high (10–100 MΩ) and so the meter must have a suitably high input impedance.

For blood pH estimation electrodes are used which enable measurement to be made with very small blood samples, or may even operate inside the body. pH meters may be used in the clinical chemistry laboratory and in intensive care areas.

Phantom r=3

Performance evaluation of radiotherapy apparatus may be conducted using a model, known as a phantom, which has properties similar to human tissue. Water demonstrates similar absorbing properties to normal tissue, and a water filled phantom may be constructed in which a radiation sensor (e.g. a small ionization chamber) may be moved to map the level of radiation at each point in the phantom. In this way the distribution of radiotherapy dose can be calculated for real treatment situations.

Phantoms are also used as teaching aids, to simulate real conditions with X-ray or ultrasonic machines. Such phantoms are also useful when setting up or calibrating imaging equipment. In nuclear medicine, phantoms are used for making absolute activity measurements.

Phased array (ultrasonic) scanner n=1 c=6 r=1

Moving picture ultrasonic B-scans can be produced by a variety of methods including rotating or rocking transducers, electronic switching of transducer elements (linear array scanners), or by electronic steering of the ultrasound beam to produce a sector scan.

Phased array scanners use a transducer with a small contact area with the skin (e.g. 1 cm by 3 cm) which can project and receive the ultrasound in a number of directions to produce a triangular image diverging from the point of contact. Inside the transducer the piezoelectric element (crystal) is divided into several parallel strips (typically 16) which are connected to the transmit pulse generator and to the receiving amplifier via a set of delay lines. If all the elements are subject to the same time delays on transmit and receive then the ultrasound beam is projected straight ahead and echoes are received from the same direction. If the left-hand end of the transducer is subject to less delay then the beam will be deflected towards the right. By progressively changing the time delay the beam may be switched or steered from left to right and back again. The electronic control over the delay lines can be improved to effect focusing of the beam on transmit, and dynamic focusing (focal length changes with time) on receive.

Such scanners are useful where the ultrasound beam must be transmitted through a small 'window' to the tissue being studied. This is particularly useful in cardiology where the heart may be viewed through a space between the ribs, or with neonates, in which case the probe is placed on top of the head before the bones have closed over. This type of scanner is relatively expensive because of its complexity.

Phonic ear

Although this is the name of a company manufacturing hearing aid equipment, the term 'phonic ear' is commonly used to describe a type of radio-frequency hearing aid for children in schools. The teacher wears a microphone/amplifier which is also a radio transmitter, and the child wears a radio receiver/hearing aid. The main advantage is that of very good signal-to-noise ratio. The teacher's voice is heard above the usual clatter and reverberation of the classroom, and the radio system allows transmission over several hundred metres (ideal for the school playing field).

Such systems are sometimes known (wrongly) as inductive loop hearing aids.

Phonic mirror n=1 c=3

This is a delayed auditory feedback machine used in the treatment of speech rhythm problems or stammering. A patient's speech may be affected (and sometimes improved) by delaying auditory feedback. The patient's voice is picked up by a microphone and fed back through headphones in a delayed and amplified form. This equipment is used in the speech therapy department.

Phonocardiograph n=2 c=4,5 r=3,9

The main sounds heard through a stethoscope placed over the heart are the noises made as the valves open and close. The first sound is low pitched, being associated with the closure of the atrio-ventricular valves and the second sound is of a higher pitch deriving from the closure of aortic and pulmonary valves. Other sounds (murmurs) indicate abnormalities.

The phonocardiograph consists of a microphone placed in a low-noise housing on the chest above the heart. The heart sounds so detected are normally split into three frequency bands and then displayed on a high-speed recorder (e.g. ultraviolet, photographic, fibre-optic, or ink jet). Diagnosis of some heart conditions can be made from a review of the phonocardiograph records having regard to the size and frequency content of the sounds, but most importantly the presence of sounds other than the main two.

The phonocardiograph is usually used in conjunction with other signals including the ECG, carotid arterial pulse, and apexcardiogram. It is sometimes used in conjunction with an echocardiograph so that the movement of the walls of the heart and valve leaflets can be represented on the same chart as the echocardiograph.

For diagnostic echocardiography, background noise can be a serious problem. The sounds are sometimes detected using a microphone mounted on a catheter passed up into the heart as part of the cardiac catheterization procedure.

Phonocatheter r=9

Phonocardiography with external microphones suffers from interference due to background noise and patient movement. Heart sounds are sometimes detected using a microphone mounted on a catheter, which is passed into the heart as part of the cardiac catheterization procedure. In fact, the miniature catheter-tip pressure transducers used within the chambers of the heart may have sufficient frequency response to collect the heart sounds as well. See also Phonocardiograph, Cardiac microphone and Cardiac catheterization equipment.

Phonophoresis apparatus r=4

A therapeutic ultrasonic treatment unit, as used in the physiotherapy department, may be used for phonophoresis to assist the passage of a drug through the skin using the ultrasonic vibrations. For example, a preparation of hydrocortisone might be applied to the skin, and the ultrasonic probe used to assist penetration by the ultrasonic massaging effect, and the local heat generated.

Photic stimulator n=1 c=4

This is a xenon flash unit designed to deliver brief flashes of light as a stimulus for electro-encephalography or for the electro-retinogram. The device consists of a photographic or strobe type of flash unit with supporting electronics to allow triggering from an external source or to operate at its own internal clock-rate and provide a trigger pulse for the recording apparatus. A photic stimulator is often included in a Ganzfeld stimulator together with other apparatus such as colour filters, fixation lights, and background illumination.

Photometer n=7 c=3,4 r=9

Although this is basically a device for measuring light intensity, in medical work it is normally associated with clinical chemistry equipment used for determining the concentration of particular chemicals in samples of body fluids. They are found in fluorimeters, spectrophotometers, colorimeters, flame photometers, atomic absorption spectrometers and in automated chemical analysers.

The basic device consists of a light-detection mechanism which uses a photomultiplier tube or semiconductor device, and this is coupled to an electronic display and recording system which may include extra components to assist in identifying the wavelengths of light involved (in this case it should be called a spectrophotometer). When used in conjunction with any of the instruments mentioned above, three extra components are required, which are a light source, a wavelength selector (which may be a filter or monochromator) to select a particular wavelength or range of wavelengths, and a sample chamber or cuvette. The light power detected by the photometer shows the amount of absorption or emission of radiation at the particular wavelength selected. By comparison with a cuvette containing a blank or calibration sample, the concentration of the test sample can be estimated.

Photomultiplier (PM) tube r=3

Photomultiplier tubes produce electric currents which are proportional to light intensity, and can detect extremely low levels of light. An important use in hospitals is in scintillation counters. In this application they detect the flashes of light occurring in a scintillation crystal due to ionizing radiation. These flashes cause the release of one or more electrons at the tube cathode and these are drawn towards the next electrode (dynode) by a high positive voltage. When these electrons strike the dynode more electrons are displaced by 'secondary emission' and they are attracted to the next dynode, and so on. By the time this sequence has been repeated several times the number of electrons is large enough to be measured. The construction of a photomultiplier tube is a series of curved dynodes (sometimes called venetian blind construction) in an evacuated glass envelope. They require a very stable high voltage supply since the output pulse height is dependent on the energy of the original radiation and on the voltage applied to the tube.

PM tubes are also used in some photometers in the pathology department.

Photoplethysmograph n=3 c=2 r=6,9

The name suggests that this device should measure volume by optical methods. In fact it is limited to detecting changes in blood perfusion in limbs and tissues. Light may be transmitted through a capillary bed such as in the ear lobe or finger tip. As arterial pulsations fill the capillary bed the changes in volume of the blood vessels modify the absorption, reflection and scattering of the light. This technique can be used to show the timing of events such as heart beats, but it is a poor measure of changes in volume and is very sensitive to motion artefacts.

A miniature tungsten lamp may be used as the light source but the heat generated causes vasodilation which alters the system being measured. An infrared light-emitting diode (LED) of a suitable colour (e.g. gallium arsenide LED) may produce a more accurate result. In their most simple form, photoplethysmographs are used for monitoring the pulse during anaesthesia or related test procedures.

Phototherapy apparatus n=5 c=3 r=4,10

This term may be applied to physiotherapy apparatus (heat lamps), but it is usually reserved for the treatment of jaundice in the newborn. For this application blue light in the range 420–500 nm oxidizes bilirubin to compounds that can more easily be eliminated from the body. The apparatus normally consists of a group of eight or ten 20–40 W fluorescent lamps spaced 30–40 cm above the unclothed infant, and fitted above the clear plastic hood of an incubator. A plastic cover on the phototherapy lamps serves as a mechanical shield and absorbs ultraviolet light. Light output in the blue range decreases with the age of the tubes and so an elapsed time meter is usually fitted to allow changing of the tubes when output begins to drop.

The infant's eyes are usually protected during this treatment, and a small probe is sometimes used to monitor the cumulative exposure.

In the physiotherapy department a range of actinotherapy schemes may be used employing light in the infrared or ultraviolet region to provide superficial heating of the tissues for relief of pain, muscle relaxation, increase of the blood supply or possibly the elimination of waste products.

Pin-index system r=2

Delivery of the wrong anaesthetic gases may cause death or permanent injury. One precaution taken to prevent this has been the introduction of an international standard system to provide non-interchangeable mating between the gas cylinder and the cylinder yokes on anaesthetic machines. This takes the form (set out in British Standard BS 1319 of 1976) of one or two pins protruding from the yoke which mate with holes in the cylinders. Pin-indexing is not used on larger cylinders or free standing cylinders for oxygen therapy.

Another precaution against the connection of incorrect cylinders is the colour coding of cylinders. Unfortunately this is not yet standardized internationally.

A similar idea has been employed to prevent the filling of anaesthetic vaporizers with the wrong agent. Examples are the Fraser Sweatman pin safety system, and the Cyprane keyed filler system which utilize non-interchangeable filling bottles and nozzles for topping up the reservoirs of anaesthetic vaporizers.

Pinkerton cuirass ventilator n=1 c=2 r=2

This is an external ventilator, which consists of a rubber bag strapped around the patient's chest, connected to a second bag which is squeezed manually to apply pressure to the chest, thus providing some artificial ventilation. Expansion of the chest is by elastic recoil. It is used in anaesthetic procedures such as bronchoscopy where access to the airways must be unobstructed.

Piped medical gas supply n=1 c=8 r=2

In larger hospitals the medical gases (and vacuum) may be supplied from a central point by pipeline. The pipeline may be supplied by banks of cylinders (usually two so that replenishing may occur without disconnection) or, in the case of oxygen, from a liquid oxygen supply. Piped supplies may consist of oxygen, nitrous oxide, Entonox, compressed air (and vacuum). The pipelines are terminated by self-closing non-interchangeable outlets in the departments where they may be used. In wards only oxygen and vacuum are normally supplied, and perhaps Entonox.

Apart from the economy of scale in providing piped supplies (the larger the gas container the lower is the unit cost) there is increased cleanliness from not having to move cylinders in and out of clean areas. Handling costs within the hospital are also reduced and there is expected to be increased reliability of supply. Shut-off valves and failure alarms are normally fitted outside the department where the supplies are used.

Piped vacuum service n=1 c=5 r=2

It is common in larger hospitals to have a central large vacuum pump and reservoir connected to a distribution network of pipes to the operating theatres and wards to operate various medical suction devices (aspirators). The pipes are terminated by self closing non-interchangeable valves similar to the piped medical gas outlets. Suction units may be plugged into these terminals to provide suction for drawing mucus and vomit from the throat and airways and possibly for wound drainage. The suction units therefore plug into the wall vacuum points and provide a variable vacuum pressure. The pipeline normally contains filters for bacteria and traps to prevent any liquid or debris from being accidentally drawn in and infecting any other parts of the system. It is usual to have two pumps and reservoirs to permit maintenance without shutdown of the system.

Pistonphone n=1 c=2

A pistonphone is an accurate and stable reference source for calibrating a sound level meter before use. The device is normally battery powered and comprises a small electric motor which drives a piston situated at one end of a small (a few millilitres) cavity into which the microphone of the sound level meter is introduced. The known and accurate excursion of the piston allows a high and constant sound pressure level to be achieved. A similar device, known as a sound level calibrator, is used for the same purpose but comprises an audio oscillator (1 kHz) and a small loudspeaker rather than a motor and piston. In addition to calibrating sound level meters they are also required for the calibration of a hearing aid test box and they are commonly found in audiology or medical physics departments.

Plan position indicator (ultrasonic) scanner r=1

A special type of ultrasonic B-scanner is available in which a small ultrasonic transducer is mounted on the side of a tube which can be passed into a natural orifice. The tube is rotated manually or by a motor such that the image is in the form of a disc representing the tissue around the tube at the level of the transducer. The most common use of this type of scanner is for visualizing the prostate gland from a site within the urethra or rectum. The probe is normally interfaced to a B-scanner which is also used for other purposes.

Plasma scalpel r=4

This is a new device for cutting and coagulating tissue achieving an effect similar to that obtained with surgical diathermy but utilizing ionized gas delivered from a nozzle under high pressure through a strong electric field. The use of an inert gas avoids chemically deleterious effects.

Plethysmograph n=5 c=2,3 r=3,9

This measures changes in volume. It may be used to measure the changes in the volume of the whole body during respiration, changes in the chest volume due to blood flow or respiration, or changes in limb volumes due to the blood flow. The common methods of measurement include electrical impedance (see Impedance plethysmograph), optical transmission or reflection changes due to blood volume changes (see Photoplethysmograph), or strain gauges may be fitted around the segment being monitored (see Mercury plethysmograph). Short-term changes in blood volume occur because the venous flow is steady whereas the arterial flow is pulsatile. Therefore the volume of the segment will vary during the cardiac cycle. Venous occlusion plethysmography is used to estimate the perfusion of a body segment by applying pressure to the proximal part of the segment to prevent the return of venous blood and then noting the rate of change of volume of the segment when the pressure is released. Sometimes the limb or limb segment is included in a chamber (chamber plethysmograph) which seals around the segment. Volume changes are calculated from the air flow in and out of the chamber, or from pressure changes.

The whole body plethysmograph, using a body box, can be used to find the residual volume (RV) of the lungs. The body box consists of a sealed chamber like a telephone box. The patient breathes through a tube to the outside and changes in chest volume are detected by changes in air pressure in the box.

Impedance plethysmography uses low-frequency alternating current which may be applied through ECG-type electrodes. This technique is used to monitor breathing and in some cases to estimate cardiac output.

Photoplethysmography utilizes the transmission or reflection of light to demonstrate the changes in blood perfusion. Such devices might be used in the cardiology department, intensive care department or for diagnostic purposes related to vascular surgery.

Pneumograph r=3,6

This is a general term for a breathing monitor, spirometer, or apnoea monitor. It is sometimes used to describe a simple chest wall movement detector utilizing a length of large-diameter tube tied around the chest and connected to a pressure transducer. The device can be used as an apnoea detector since the pressure in the tube will vary continually unless breathing ceases. This type of apnoea detector is unlikely to be found now. Electrical pneumographs also exist using mercury-in-rubber strain gauges wound around the chest or using electrical impedance measurements across the thorax.

Pneumotachometer/graph n=3 c=4 r=3,6,9

This measures the flow rate of gases during breathing. The breath is passed through a short tube (Fleisch tube) in which there is a fine mesh which presents a small resistance to the flow. The resulting pressure drop across the mesh is in proportion to the flow rate. The pressure drop is very small (e.g. 2 mmHg) and so the measuring circuit must be of high quality and produce very little drift with time. A differential pressure transducer is normally used.

The advantage which this device has over the mechanical spirometer is that the patient under investigation can continue to breathe fresh air through the transducer while the measurements are taken. The volume in each breath and the cumulative volume can be found by electronic integration of the flow rate. Problems exist because inspired and expired volumes and gas mixtures are not the same, and so the pressure drop will not be the same for equal flow in each direction. Also, water vapour in the expired gases may condense on the mesh unless heating is applied, or some other anti-condensation measure is used.

The pneumotachograph may be used in lung function analysis, or during artificial ventilation of the lungs. For routine work in each of these applications simpler devices are normally used, such as the spirometer, dry gas meter, and the Wright's respirometer or Wright's respiration meter.

Polarographic cell r=4

Measurement of oxygen concentration may be achieved using a special cell covered with an oxygen permeable membrane (usually PTFE – Teflon). A tiny platinum cathode beneath the membrane is maintained at approximately 0.6 V with respect to a reference electrode of silver-silver chloride to select the oxygen, and the current produced is linearly proportional to the oxygen partial pressure. Such devices may be used to measure oxygen concentration in gases for monitoring during anaesthetic and oxygen therapy procedures or they may be used for determining oxygen tension in blood samples, blood within the body or through the skin.

The electrodes are relatively slow acting and do not last indefinitely. The cell is sometimes known as the Clark electrode.

Polygraph n=5 c=4,5

This is simply a multichannel pen recorder with a set of special preamplifiers (signal conditioning units) so that a number of physiological signals can be recorded simultaneously. The term usually applies to pen recorders but could equally be used to describe ultraviolet, ink-jet, or photographic recorders. Typical signals monitored using a polygraph might be arterial or other pressures, skin resistance, temperature, etc. The term 'polygraph' is sometimes used in popular works to mean 'lie detector', which is a skin resistance meter used for non-medical purposes.

Pop-off valve r=2

A common name given to an expiratory valve used in anaesthetic breathing circuits. The expiratory valve is a form of pressure relief valve to release the gases which are breathed out.

Potassium ion analyser n=5 c=4

Measurement of the concentration of potassium ions in whole blood or plasma may be made by using an ion selective electrode which is sensitive to potassium ions. The voltage between the potassium ion electrode and a reference electrode is proportional to the potassium ion concentration in the sample. This technique is used in both stat (discrete sample) analysers, and autoanalysers in chemical pathology laboratories and intensive care units. It may be a separate instrument or combined with (for example) a sodium ion meter.

Potentiometric recorder n=20 c=3,4 r=3

Slow-moving variables such as trends of pressure, heart rate or output from analytical instruments in the pathology laboratory may be recorded on wide paper using a potentiometric recorder, usually in the flat-bed format. The pen is mounted on a wire which moves it across the width of the recording paper with the aid of pulleys driven by a motor. One of the pulleys is mounted on the spindle of a potentiometer (although this can be a single length of resistance wire) which generates a voltage output proportional to the position of the pen. This voltage is applied to the input of the amplifier which drives the motor, as a negative feedback signal, so that the pen is always moved to a point corresponding to the amplitude of the input signal to be recorded. Preamplifiers are added to scale and condition the signal according to its amplitude, frequency content, and type (e.g. differential).

The writing speed is determined by the power of the motor, mass of the moving system (wires pulleys and pens) so that the pen has a maximum acceleration and velocity. The system is attractive where wide paper is desired and where high linearity is required (e.g. 0.2%). The system is unsuitable for fast moving signals or where multichannel operation is required. Multichannel systems exist but different colours are needed and there must be a small offset between each pen to avoid them colliding. X-Y recorders are usually potentiometric.

Potter-Bucky diaphragm r=7

More commonly known as a 'Bucky', this is an assembly which is normally located under the table of a diagnostic X-ray set and holds the X-ray film cassette and the secondary radiation grid. The grid is used to prevent secondary X-ray emission from the patient from reaching the X-ray film, and is formed from a large number of thin strips of lead separated by a radiolucent material. To prevent the outline of the grid from appearing on the film a mechanism is provided for moving the grid during exposure. The Bucky is mounted on bearings which permit movement along rails under the X-ray table so that the grid and film can be moved to an appropriate position under the patient. The Bucky is used with most diagnostic X-ray equipment.

Vertical, pedestal, and cantilever types exist which can be used with mobile X-ray sets. For ward and theatre work, stationary grids are sometimes used with ordinary cassettes, or the grid is within the cassette.

Pressure regulator r=2

These are used in very large numbers in medical gas supplies. Their function is to reduce the pressure of cylinder or piped gases to a working level (usually 4 or 7 bar), or to a low pressure suitable for breathing. They consist of a valve on the high-pressure supply which is linked to a diaphragm on the low-pressure side. Variations on the low-pressure side (for instance due to flow rate changes) will cause the high-pressure valve to adjust to give the correct flow to keep the low pressure correct. Various types exist such as the Adams regulator but those used on cylinders are usually two stage (i.e. there is an intermediate stage of pressure reduction) since this gives a more stable low-pressure output with widely varying demands on gas flow.

Pressure relief valve r=2

To release excess gases or pressure from a closed circuit, these are used in many kinds of apparatus and are commonly encountered in anaesthetic apparatus. Pressure can be limited to a safe level by setting a pressure relief valve to allow gas to escape freely if the set pressure is exceeded. They may also be used to regulate pressure (rather wastefully), by releasing excess gas so that the relief valve is open all the time.

Pressure transducer n=30 r=3,9

Physiological pressures range from about 18 kPa (140 mmHg) for arterial blood pressure to 0.26 kPa (2mmHg) for airways pressure. These and other pressures may be measured and recorded for diagnostic or monitoring purposes. Because the mercury manometer is used so much for blood pressure recording it is very common to quote physiological pressure in millimetres of mercury (mmHg) rather than in SI units (Pa – pascals). Also some pressures such as bladder pressure and central venous pressure are often quoted in centimetres of water head. This is particularly convenient with water-filled measurement tubing since changes in the height of the transducer or patient make the same changes in the measured pressure. Useful conversions are as follows:

1 mmHg = 133 Pa = 0.133 kPa
1 mmHg = 1.36 cmH$_2$O
1 cmH$_2$O = 0.735 mmHg

Although static pressures can be measured using a column of mercury (e.g. the mercury sphygmomanometer) or water, changing pressures require a pressure transducer which can respond to rapid changes. These usually work by producing an electrical signal from the bending of a membrane or diaphragm. The strain gauge which measures the bending may be part of the pressure diaphragm itself as in semiconductor gauges or it may be attached to the diaphragm (usually a thin steel plate) by a rod. The strain gauges change their electrical resistance as the diaphragm is bent by the pressure. The gauges form part of a bridge circuit which provides a voltage output corresponding to the applied pressure. A differential amplifier is required to amplify this signal before delivery to a CRT monitor or pen recorder. Inductive, capacitance, and piezoelectric strain gauges also exist.

Physiological pressure transducers are usually 2–3 cm in diameter and are mounted in a clamp close to the patient and connected to the site of measurement (artery, heart, bladder, lungs etc.) by a narrow tube which is usually filled with water or saline. Special miniature versions also exist which are mounted on the tip of a narrow tube which can be passed directly into the body.

Favourable characteristics for a pressure transducer are high-frequency response, low drift with temperature and time, low compliance, and electrical isolation.

Proctoscope

This is a general term for an instrument for passing through the anus to examine the lower rectum. It is a straight tube, often with a small light bulb mounted at the end. The sigmoidoscope is a longer version of the same instrument. Disposable proctoscopes, without light, are also available.

Profilometer n=1 c=4

Although this term could have other meanings, in medical equipment it usually refers to a device for recording the profile of urethral closure pressure along its length. The apparatus consists of a catheter puller, to draw a pressure measuring catheter along the length of the urethra, and a mechanism to record the urethral wall pressure. This may be a tiny pressure transducer mounted on the side or tip of the recording catheter, or an external pressure transducer linked via tubing to a side hole in the urethral catheter through which a small (e.g. 2 ml/min) flow of water or saline is maintained.

The apparatus may be self contained or incorporated into a general urodynamic test set. Such devices are found in the urology, gynaecology, or X-ray department.

Progressive treatment unit $r=10$

This is another name for an electrotherapy apparatus used in the physiotherapy department for exercising denervated or wasted muscles by passing electric current through the tissues from surface or internal electrodes, or electrodes in a water bath. The currents may be interrupted direct current, low-frequency alternating current (e.g. 50 Hz) or faradic currents. The unit normally has controls to vary the intensity and the duration of the treatment pulses and can cause them to rise in a progressive manner throughout the treatment with periods of rest between the groups of pulses to enable the muscles to recover.

Proportioning pump

This mixes two fluids in a fixed ratio, and is found in a haemodialysis machine for mixing a concentrated solution with treated tap water to produce the dialysate. It usually consists of a motorized pump with a double chamber in which the relative volumes of the two chambers can be adjusted to provide the correct mixing proportions.

Proportioning pumps are also used in some laboratory apparatus to achieve exact dilutions of samples of body fluids before passing to an analyser.

Prosthesis $r=4$

Medical devices used to replace lost or absent function are called prosthetic devices or prostheses. The structure of a prosthesis may not resemble the natural element since its main intention is to replace function. Artificial heart valves and artificial hips are examples of prostheses.

Pulse duplicator $r=4$

This term is used to describe a heart simulator for investigating the flow characteristics of blood within the heart, particularly for evaluating the performance of artificial heart valves. Flow conditions are simulated in a Perspex model made from a mould of the inside of a cadaver heart and a blood-equivalent mixture is pumped with a pressure cycle similar to that found in normal conditions. Artificial heart valves may be mounted at the normal sites in the model and flow may be monitored using high-speed photography of small particles suspended in the fluid. Pressure measurements may also be recorded.

Such devices would only be found in a cardiac research laboratory.

Pulse height analyser n=3 c=3 r=3

The amplitudes of pulses from a scintillation detector used in nuclear medicine vary according to the energy of the incident rays. A pulse height analyser is an electronic device employed to identify those pulses falling between two preset amplitude levels which may relate only to the product of a single isotope. This process is sometimes called window discrimination. A number of pulse height analysers may be operated in parallel and the results collected by a multichannel analyser to show count rates from a number of isotopes simultaneously.

Another type of pulse height analyser is used to plot the size distribution of blood cells in conjunction with a cell counter.

Pulse monitor n=30 c=1 r=2

A simple device to indicate that a peripheral pulse exists and is regular. It may operate from a microphone over a palpable artery, a pressure bulb taped to the skin, or by photoelectric transmission or reflection at the finger tip or ear lobe. A simple monitor would probably be battery operated and contain a detector circuit, and a meter on which the needle kicks in time to the pulse, or a light or bleep is activated on each pulse. They may also include a ratemeter. These devices are mainly used by anaesthetists.

Pulse rate meter n=10 c=2 r=2

This is an extension of the simple pulse monitor, and is a device used by anaesthetists to monitor pulse rate. The pulse is detected and averaged from a microphone over an artery, a pressure bulb taped on to the skin, or a photo-electric device detecting the fluctuations in the red light transmitted through or reflected from a finger or ear lobe due to the pulse.

Pulsed wave doppler ultrasonic flowmeter n=1 c=5 r=9

Ultrasonic flowmeters can be used to measure and record instantaneous blood flow from outside the body, employing an ultrasound beam transmitted through the skin. Most are continuous wave (CW) flowmeters which provide little information about the flow profile, and so pulsed instruments have been developed which can identify the flow velocity at any point beneath the probe. The size and depth of the measurement point can be varied by adjusting the pulse length and timing of the range-gate. By examining the doppler shift at various depths we may obtain a velocity profile across a blood vessel. Typical parameters for this device would be an ultrasonic frequency of 8 MHz, pulse duration of 1 μs (which produces a travelling packet of sound 1.5 mm long), and pulse repetition frequency of 10 000 c/s.

The blood velocities recorded from each point across the profile can be displayed separately on a chart recorder after analysis by zero-crossing detector, and these signals may be combined to produce a figure for blood flow rate through the vessels. However, there are many variations on the end processing of pulsed wave doppler signals and these are not covered here.

Since range information is available as well as information about blood flow it is possible to combine it with an ultrasonic B-scan display (two-dimensional section of tissue) so that the point at which the measurement is being made in the tissue can be identified and manipulated. In more complex instruments a 'doppler scan' can be produced which is a B-scan, but showing only the moving parts of the picture (blood flow in arteries).

Pump r=2,3,4

Various types of pump are found in medical work. Some of the types and terms used are given below:

1. Blood pump. In haemodialysis and during open heart surgery blood is pumped round an extracorporeal (outside the body) circuit by roller pumps. Blood may also be pumped for blood transfusion, but this is less common.
2. Syringe pump. A syringe may be mounted on a motorized track which squeezes the syringe slowly to infuse drugs into the body in a controlled manner. Spring-loaded syringes are also used in some applications.
3. Vacuum pump. These are the basis of all suction pumps used throughout the hospital for sucking accumulated liquids from wounds and inside the nasopharynx and lungs. These may be small portable units or central plant maintaining a vacuum throughout a piped distribution network. They are also used in ultrafiltration apparatus.
4. Respirable air pump. A clean source of breathing air is sometimes produced with a pump and filter to be used in anaesthetic applications.
5. Infusion pump. This is a widely used term covering peristaltic, motorized syringe, and sometimes infusion controllers which do not strictly have a pumping action. They are used throughout hospitals in large numbers for the controlled intravenous infusion of drugs and other fluids.

6. Volumetric infusion pump. This describes a reciprocating syringe type of pump used for the infusion of drugs in the ward and in operating theatre. These are said to be more accurate in the quantities delivered than peristaltic infusion pumps which normally rely on the counting of drops falling in the drip chamber in the infusion set. Errors in the counting of drops due to damage, misuse or faulty apparatus are potentially dangerous.
7. Implantable or ambulatory drug pumps. Small electric, clockwork or pneumatic infusion pumps may be carried on the person or implanted. Such pumps are becoming increasingly important for long-term therapy where a hospital stay would be unnecessary and expensive.
8. Dialysis pump. This is a proportioning pump to mix a concentrated dialysing fluid with purified tap water to produce a mixture of controlled concentration in a haemodialysis machine.

Pupillometer

This is a device for measuring the size and changes in size of the pupil of the eye. Various methods have been used. None are in common use.

Pure tone audiometer n=5 c=4 r=3,8

Although a true test of hearing ability would have to include a test of comprehension of the spoken word, a simpler test to find the patient's threshold of hearing at several standard frequencies is more practical and usually sufficient to direct the course of treatment. Thus most audiometric tests involve the presentation of tones of increasing or decreasing intensity to establish the level at which the patient first becomes aware of the sounds (hearing threshold). A pure tone audiometer generates tones throughout the audible range (usually at each octave between 125 Hz and 8 kHz) at amplitudes related to the expected thresholds for a normally hearing person. The difference between the patient threshold and the normal (i.e. the hearing loss) is expressed in decibels (dBHL) and recorded on an audiogram chart.

The tones are usually presented to the patient through headphones, but a loudspeaker can be used, although this is less precise. If there is a large difference between the hearing loss occurring at each ear (greater than 40 dB) then a masking tone must be introduced to the better ear while the test tones are presented to the other. Having established the hearing loss using the air-conduction methods as above, the procedure is usually repeated using bone conduction to determine whether the same loss is recorded when the inner ear is stimulated directly.

A diagnostic audiometer consists of a signal generator producing tones and masking noises, with calibrated scales of frequency and amplitude, and capable of driving headphones or bone conduction transducers. A simpler (screening) type of audiometer is often used in schools and health centres. This does not normally have a bone conduction facility, but may be fitted with special noise-excluding headphones.

PUVA skin treatment apparatus $n=1$ $c=4$ $r=10$

Irradiation with ultraviolet light in the UVA part of the spectrum (280-400 nm) is sometimes performed in conjunction with a photo-active drug such as Psoralen as Psoralen ultraviolet A treatment (PUVA). The apparatus for this is a form of tunnel bath employing banks of fluorescent UVA tubes arranged inside a reflector around the patient. Periods of skin treatment may be typically 2 hours at a time and this may be undertaken in the physiotherapy department, or in the skin clinic.

R

Radiant heat lamp n=5 c=2 r=10

These radiate long wavelength infrared rays to produce superficial heating either in the treatment of inflammation (physiotherapy department) or as a substitute for an enclosed canopy incubator to keep small babies warm during observation and treatment. The lamps may be incandescent filament lamps with a special glass filter to reduce visible and ultraviolet radiation or they may be non-visible, employing overwound or enclosed heating elements of the type used in domestic electric heaters.

Radiation pressure (force) balance n=1 c=3 r=1

Radiation (waves) exerts a force on objects which reflect or absorb it. The effect can be used to measure the power of an ultrasonic beam by directing it on to a reflector coupled to a force measuring device. The forces involved are very small (0.135 mg/mW) and so the measurement device must be extremely sensitive. There are various designs, including a reflector suspended by fine wires which moves in response to the ultrasound radiation in a water bath, a reflector made in the form of a float which is pushed downwards, or the reflector may be the face of a strain gauge pressure transducer. Such devices would be found in the physics or electronics laboratory for calibrating or testing the output of ultrasonic devices.

Radiation thermometer r=9

There is a known relationship between the surface temperature of an object and its radiant power. This principle makes it possible to measure the temperature of a body without physical contact with it. Medical thermography is a technique whereby the temperature distribution of the surface of the body is mapped within a few tenths of a kelvin. The human skin approximates to within 1% of a black body radiator and so a radiation thermometer can accurately detect the temperature of the skin. The detector in a radiation thermometer is typically arsenic trisulphide, indium antimonide, lead sulphide or thallium bromide iodine. The actual detector used will depend on the wavelengths (usually in the far infrared) required to be detected. Most thermography apparatus employs a mirror-type focusing

210

device and the radiation beam is fed to the detector through a chopping disc which has a slot in it to interrupt the beam at a frequency of several hundred hertz so that an a.c. amplifier and phase sensitive detector can be used to amplify without the drift associated with d.c. amplifiers. See also Thermography apparatus.

Radio pill

This is a radio transmitter, small enough to be swallowed, which may operate from inside the body. It transmits electrical, pressure, or pH signals from within the gut. Similar devices can be introduced into the bladder to record pressure changes. They are usually epoxy encapsulated and contain a simple Hartley oscillator circuit operating at low frequency (e.g. 0.5 MHz) which is detected outside the body with a loop aerial. More complex devices are possible which may be implanted, but these are not often used clinically.

Radiotherapy equipment n=3 c=6,7 r=3

Ionizing radiation may be used as therapy since tumour cells are more susceptible to radiation damage than normal cells. The radiation used may be X-rays, beta-rays (electrons), gamma-rays, alpha particles, or neutron beams.

The effect is to displace electrons from atoms, thereby causing disruption of cell chemistry. The radiation dose which reaches the tumour depends upon the distance between the source and the skin, how well the radiation penetrates the tissues, and the quantity of radiation scattered into the treatment area from surrounding tissues. The depth of penetration of the radiation increases as the energy of the source increases and treatment is therefore provided for superficial tumours using low voltage X-rays (15–150 kV) and much higher energies (e.g.15 MeV) using an accelerator for deep-seated tumours.

Teletherapy apparatus produces radiation beams outside the body and directs them through the skin, varying the point of entry to the body to reduce the average dose at the skin if the area to be treated is deep within the body. Alternatively, sealed radioactive sources may be placed within body cavities to provide localized radiotherapy in a particular organ.

Radiotherapy is a complex subject, usually conducted in a special department employing doctors expert in cancer treatment, radiographers (therapy), physicists for treatment planning and dose calculations and technicians to manage the apparatus.

Radium needle r=3

This is a small needle or rod usually made of platinum or iridium alloys and containing a few milligrams of a radioactive substance such as radium or caesium-137. The device is shaped as a needle so that it can be inserted into the tissue to provide localized radiotherapy. At one end is a small hole through which a thread is passed so that the device can be withdrawn. In a typical treatment a number of needles may be inserted in a configuration to provide the best pattern of radiation to the tumour to be treated with minimal radiation beyond.

A larger quantity of radioactive material may be included in a radium tube where the whole device can be inserted into a body space. Such devices are used in the radiotherapy department.

Radium tube r=3

Localized radiotherapy may be delivered within the body by insertion of a small metal tube (often silver) containing a quantity of radium or caesium-137. Such tubes are used in the radiotherapy or oncology department.

Range-gated doppler ultrasonic flowmeter r=9

The flow velocity at various points across a blood vessel can be obtained from outside the body using a pulsed wave doppler ultrasonic flowmeter. These employ range-gating by which the flow velocity can be measured at a relatively well-defined point (e.g. within 2 mm) and at any distance from the transducer along the line of the transmitted ultrasound beam. Such devices may produce information about the flow pattern at a particular point within an artery or may be used to produce a velocity profile. They can also be combined with B-scanners to identify the sampling point on the B-scan image, or used to present a special B-scan image on which only the rapidly moving parts (blood within the arteries) are shown. See also Pulsed wave doppler ultrasonic velocity meter.

Reaction rate analyser n=1 c=5,6 r=9

This is used for determining concentration of enzymes in samples of body fluids. Most chemical determinations are made using the end point of a chemical reaction, and the concentrations are established by photometric methods. In the case of enzymes the concentrations are manifested through the rate of a particular chemical reaction. Thus the progress of the reaction must be monitored throughout its course so that the reaction rate either at the beginning of the reaction or during the course of it can be determined by curve fitting or some other method, usually by computer.

One particular type of reaction rate analyser is the centrifugal autoanalyser in which the reactions take place in cuvettes mounted around the edge of a centrifuge rotor which passes between the light source and the photometer of a colorimeter. The progress of the reaction taking place in each cuvette can be monitored at frequent intervals determined by the speed of the rotor. The initial or standard reaction rate may be determined to identify the concentration of an enzyme. The standard rate of reaction may be used to determine such enzymes as alkaline phosphatase, creatinine phosphokinase, lactate dehydrogenase, serum glutamic oxaloacetic transaminase, and serum pyruvic transaminase. An enzyme analyser is usually a reaction rate analyser.

Real-time ultrasonic scanner $n=5$ $c=6$ $r=1$

This is an ultrasonic scanner which produces a moving picture at the time of scanning. The expression 'real-time' is an unfortunate use of a computer term which relates to the immediate processing and presentation of information, so that for practical purposes the results are available straight away. Real-time scanners have been available since the mid 1960s, but they did not become popular until about 1976 when a range of new types of scanner was introduced. These include linear array scanners, electronic sector scanners, rocking and rotating transducer types, and moving mirror scanners. Most impact has been made by those with no moving parts. The picture quality with most real-time scanners appears inferior to the classical hand operated B-scanner but it now appears that the overall information gained by the operator is greater using the new types of scanner, partly due to the more positive appreciation of the scanning plane, but mostly due to the extra prompts and landmarks provided by moving structures which enable better identification of organs.

The most common form of real-time scanner is the linear array scanner in which a large hand-held transducer is applied to the skin with a contact area of about 1 cm by 10 cm. The piezo electric element (crystal) in the transducer is divided into many parallel elements and these are connected in groups so that an active area is commutated along from one end to the other. The picture produced is in the form of a rectangle whose upper short edge corresponds to the face of the transducer. The long edge is the length of the ultrasonic scan line. Apart from the transducer control mechanism, which is wholly electronic, the apparatus need be no more complicated than an A-scanner. Modern types of real-time scanner usually include a frame freeze module by which every point on the picture is stored in a computer memory and can therefore be held on the screen for examination or photography.

Most real-time scanners only perform a 'simple' scan in that each point in the tissue is only interrogated from a single direction.

Rebreathing bag $n=300$ $c=1$ $r=2$

This is physically the same as a reservoir bag, both being used in anaesthesia.

Typical size is 2 litres. The usual function of the rebreathing bag is to act as a reservoir for the expired (and then rebreathed) gases in a rebreathing circuit or to be the instrument for propelling gases into the lungs during assisted ventilation. They are usually made in black antistatic rubber with a wide bore connector at the top.

Rebreathing circuit r=2

In anaesthesia, exhaled gases may be discarded, and new gases inspired from the anaesthetic machine, or the same gases may be re-inhaled, totally or in part. Full rebreathing as occurs in a closed (e.g. circle) circuit needs a carbon dioxide absorber. Partial rebreathing as in a semi-closed circuit (e.g. Magill) may not use an absorber. Rebreathing circuits are economical with the gases and vapours, cause little air pollution, and are more suitable for use with assisted ventilation.

Rectilinear scanner n=3 c=5,6 r=3

This is a large scintillation counter with collimator which is moved over the body in a rectilinear motion so as to map the distribution of radioactivity. It is used in the nuclear medicine or X-ray department to investigate the distribution of radionuclides following the administration of a radiophar-maceutical. The best known example of its use is in scanning for the distribution of iodine uptake by the thyroid gland. The results are plotted using a dotting recorder, or a computer image is formed.

Rees T-piece paediatric circuit r=2

Most anaesthetics are delivered via a Magill attachment of the breathing circuit components. This unfortunately produces resistance to expiration due to the use of an expiratory valve. In paediatrics this is often avoided by the use of a T-piece circuit in which a length of breathing tube is used as a reservoir for the exhaled gases and for fresh gas. This is unsatisfactory if assisted ventilation is required since no pressure can be developed within the circuit. The Rees circuit overcomes this problem by the use of a double-ended reservoir bag at the free end of the breathing tube. Ventilation is assisted by squeezing the bag while closing the open end of the bag between a finger and thumb. The finger is released during the expiratory phase.

Regulator r=2

These are common components in the delivery system for medical gases, particularly for cylinder oxygen supplies. A regulator will consist of a high-pressure valve operated by a diaphragm on the low-pressure side. Variations in the low-pressure output will be compensated for by suitable automatic adjustments in the flow rate of the high-pressure gas. Cooling fins may be provided to prevent icing due to the Joule–Thomson effect, as in the Adams regulator.

Many gas regulators are two-stage regulators which provide a more stable low-pressure output in widely varying flow conditions.

Regulators often have integral pressure gauges to show the performance of input and output pressures.

Relaxometer n=1 c=2,3

This helps the subject to reduce his level of autonomic arousal. It produces an audible signal whose pitch varies with the level of activity in the autonomic nervous system. Skin resistance is measured with two simple surface electrodes and translated into a continuous tone. Excitement causes a drop in skin resistance and a rise in the pitch of the tone. When the subject hears the pitch drop he knows that he is relaxing. This can be a bench instrument or a pocket-worn device used with an ear plug. Such devices may sometimes be used in the speech therapy department.

Reservoir bag n=300 c=1 r=2

This is a rubber bag used during gas anaesthesia to store fresh gases supplied from the continuous flow anaesthetic machine during the expiratory phase, and to deliver this gas (or part of it) during inspiration. It is physically identical to a rebreathing bag, and a normal adult bag has a 2 litre capacity. It may be used to assist ventilation of the patient's lungs by squeezing it during inspiration. Normally the bag is soft and floppy so that it does not apply significant pressure to the lungs. A stiffer bag may be used with some ventilators on which the bag plays a part in the action (e.g. Autovent). Some ventilators may require a special pressure-limiting bag from which gas is automatically vented when it fills beyond a certain amount. Should the bag overfill, the elasticity of the bag itself will limit the final pressure.

Reservoir bags are normally single ended (e.g. for attachment to the bag mount on the anaesthetic machine) but can be double ended such as for use in the Rees T-piece paediatric circuit. In this case ventilation is assisted by squeezing the bag while sealing the bag outlet tube with a finger, and then releasing this for the rest of the breathing cycle.

Respirable air pump n=2 c=3

A clean air source, free from oil, dust, or other debris, is required to drive

215

lung ventilators where there is no piped medical air supply. A respirable air pump may have an inlet for oxygen together with flowmeters for air and oxygen to give accurate monitoring of minute volume output of an air/oxygen mixture. The Blease respirable air pump also has a safety valve set at 5 psi and the oxygen supply pressure should be 60 psi.

Respirator r=2

This is a device for artificial ventilation of the lungs, also known as a resuscitator. The term is normally applied to an emergency apparatus consisting of a self-inflating bag, valves, and face mask, perhaps with provision for an oxygen supply. Common types are the Ambu, Air Viva, Cardiff inflating bellows, Oxford inflating bellows and the Samson infant resuscitator.

Respirometer n=30 c=2 r=2

It is useful to measure the volume or flow rate of gases entering or leaving the lungs during anaesthesia, particularly if assisted ventilation is being used. The best known device for this is the Wright's respirometer which can be fitted into the breathing circuit and works by directing the gases on to a rotating vane which drives a gear train attached to a pointer moving over a dial. It only measures gas movement in one direction because the forward flow is directed on to the vanes through oblique slots in a small drum surrounding the vane. Retrograde flow enters the device along the axis of the vane.

Retinoscope

This is similar to the ophthalmoscope, and is used to examine the interior of the eye under direct observation. The aim is to obtain an index of the refractive qualities of the patient's lens system. It generates and optically processes a narrow high-intensity rotatable light beam which passes through the subject's lenses in order to give a full, sharp, clear reflex image without any peephole shadow.

Resuscitator r=2

This term is usually applied to an apparatus for emergency ventilation of the lungs, and may also be called a respirator. It normally refers to a self-inflating air bag, valves and a face mask, perhaps with provision for an oxygen supply. Examples are the Ambu, Air Viva, Cardiff inflating bellows, Oxford inflating bellows and the Samson infant resuscitator.

A defibrillator may also sometimes be called a resuscitator.

Reverse osmosis machine n=10 c=3,4,5 r=3

Water will pass through a semipermeable membrane from the weaker solution to the stronger solution. If sufficient pressure is applied to the stronger solution (in excess of the osmotic pressure) water can be made to pass in the opposite direction. This is reverse osmosis.

The technique is used in industry for producing pure water and is of interest in the production of sterile water for medical work such as for solutions for irrigating the bladder, for dialysis, and potentially for intravenous fluids. The cost of pure sterile water produced by this method is cheaper than the alternatives which normally involve distillation and autoclaving. Equipment is already available to produce water for bladder irrigation, and for haemodialysis. Production of water for haemodialysis by reverse osmosis is desirable where the tap water used to make up the dialysate solution contains excessive amounts of aluminium compounds.

The equipment consists of filters, water softeners or de-ionizers, carbon filter, and a semipermeable membrane driven on the input side at a high pressure. The process may be supplemented by autoclaving, boiling or pasteurizing before use.

Ripple bed/mattress n=20 c=2

Patients who are immobile for long periods may develop pressure sores. These can be avoided by repeatedly moving the patient so that different parts of the skin are supporting the body weight. An alternative method is to use a ripple mattress in which different segments of the mattress are repeatedly inflated and deflated to vary the positions where pressure is applied to the skin. There are two types of these, water-filled and air-filled types. The water-filled types are also used to provide heat and are much thinner (see Heated ripple mattress).

The air-filled types may have large or small inflatable cells and there are cushions and seats which use the same principle. The air pump inflates and deflates the alternative cells over a period of a few minutes (e.g. 10 minutes). The controller unit includes a small pump and valves to control the delivery between two or more circuits in the mattress. One trade name for these is the Pulsair mattress.

Rocking apparatus

Respiration can be assisted by rocking the patient so that the weight of the abdominal contents moves the diaphragm up and down. Special rocking beds have been made for this.

217

Roller pump n=30 c=2,3

To preserve sterility of body fluids (e.g. blood) during pumping they can be pumped inside soft rubber tubes squeezed between rollers. The rollers move forward keeping a part of the tube closed. This produces a pulsatile or peristaltic form of flow which is suitable for many applications such as pumping during haemodialysis and open-heart surgery. The usual form has two or three rollers on a rotating arm which presses the tubing into a shoe so that one of the rollers is always occluding the tube (thus preventing back flow). The tubing must be relatively soft. It may be part of a long silicon-rubber tube or it may be a short section within a stiffer tube. This type of pump produces relatively little damage to blood.

A modified form of roller pump is used in many automatic infusion pumps. A set of cams drive a row of fingers which squeeze the tube in turn, so that the closed point moves forward. As the last finger closes on the tube the first one will seal the tube to prevent back flow, and the process is repeated. See also Blood pump, and Heart-lung machine.

Rotameter r=2

This is a trade name which is commonly used for a type of flowmeter which is in widespread use for medical gases. It consists of a vertical glass or plastic tube which has an internal taper narrowing towards the bottom. Gases are fed in through a needle valve at the base and flow rate is metered as the height to which a bobbin rises up the tube. The bobbin is designed to rotate in the flowing gas so that it does not stick or oscillate and can be seen to be moving freely. Because of the different physical properties of each gas, a differently calibrated rotameter is required.

A continuous-flow anaesthetic machine has three, four, or five rotameters, and they are also found in the wards and clinics on oxygen therapy apparatus. To perform correctly they must be vertical in use. Errors can also arise due to static electricity on the glass, and they may stick if there is any dirt in the tube. Thus, servicing usually includes an annual cleaning and leak test.

Ruben's valve c=1 r=2

This is an expiratory valve for use in non-rebreathing anaesthetic circuits. It is a two-stage valve intended to improve on the performance of the single-disc expiratory valves (e.g. Heidbrink), in that all the exhaled gases are vented to atmosphere, and excess fresh gas is also vented. The dead space is thus reduced. It consists of two spring-loaded disc valves.

S

Salt valve c=1 r=2

A type of expiratory valve used in anaesthesia. This particular valve has no spring in order to minimize resistance but has a simple closure mechanism for use in controlled ventilation.

Scan converter r=1

This is a device to change the scanning system of a video (e.g. TV) signal. They were developed for converting television recordings made in one country for showing in another, but are used in medical ultrasound scanners to convert the ultrasound scanning system to a TV video format. There are two main types of scan converter.

The analogue type takes the form of a television tube and television camera tube connected end to end so that an image written on to a screen between the two sections of the tube can be presented at one line and frame rate, and read off by the camera portion of the tube at a different rate. The image is not actually formed as a visible image but is merely an electrostatic image on a silicon plate.

The second, and now more common type, is the digital scan converter which has a large computer memory having one memory location for every picture element (pixel). The memory is written to, and read from, at the two different scan rates.

A major drawback with early ultrasonic B-scanners lay in the image storage mechanism. Bi-stable storage cathode ray tubes were used which could only produce a line image (i.e. black and white with no intermediate shades). Since part of the diagnostic information is contained in the differing amplitudes of the echoes from different tissues, the inability to display this as variations in brightness meant that there was some loss of diagnostic information. The analogue scan converter solved this problem since it could produce an image of wide dynamic range (low contrast) which could be frozen.

It has since been found that scan converters are also useful with moving picture scanners to provide a 'frame freeze' facility. The moving image can be frozen at will, or according to a synchronizing signal (e.g. ECG) and the resulting still picture can be photographed or measurements taken. The digital scan converters have completely supplanted the analogue types for this work because of their stability and flexibility. Being computer compatible, supplementary programs can be run to produce image improvements, area measurements, and alpha-numeric information on the display. Scan converters usually produce a television-type signal which can be viewed on one or more monitors and can be recorded on videotape.

Scavenging system r=2

It is desirable to remove gases exhaled by patients in operating theatres because of the effects of the anaesthetic agents on the staff. The mechanism of removal of these gases has become known as scavenging. Scavenging systems include long breathing tubes on the expiratory port to carry the gases to the extraction side of the air-conditioning system, or to a special low-grade suction system ducting the gases outside the building. Halothane can be removed by connection to a special activated charcoal absorber (see Aldasorber).

Schimmelbusch mask n=50 c=1 r=2

Ether and chloroform can be administered directly on to a gauze or lint in front of a patient's mouth to induce anaesthesia. The Schimmelbusch mask is a proprietary mask to facilitate the inhalation of these agents. It may be supplied in a modified form to permit the delivery of one or more anaesthetic gases at the same time.

Scintillation camera n=2 c=6

This is another name for a gamma camera. It usually consists of a large sodium iodide crystal and a collimator arranged so that radioactivity within an organ causes scintillations within the crystal at points corresponding to the position of radionuclides within the organ. The positions are calculated by computer from the light flashes (scintillations) detected by an array of photomultiplier (PM) tubes positioned above the crystal. The device is used in the nuclear medicine or X-ray department for producing images of the distribution of radionuclides in the organs under investigation.

Scintillation counter n=5 r=3

A scintillation counter is the ionizing radiation detection system used in gamma cameras and isotope scanners, and in some pathology laboratory apparatus. It consists of a scintillator (usually a sodium iodide crystal), a photomultiplier (PM) tube, and supporting electronics. Scintillators glow when exposed to X-rays and small flashes occur in response to gamma rays. Thus an electric pulse can be generated by the photomultiplier tube for each gamma-ray interaction.

This system is employed in the gamma camera and rectilinear scanner, to produce a map of radionuclide distribution within the body. The scintillation count, or count rate, indicates the quantity of a radiopharmaceutical, and the intensity of the scintillation indicates the energy of the rays.

In the pathology laboratory a scintillation counter may be used to identify the concentration of radio-labelled chemicals. In some cases a liquid scintillator may be used.

Screening audiometer n=5 c=2 r=3

The simplest form of pure tone audiometer consists of a portable unit which delivers a few (e.g. four) different tone frequencies at a restricted range of intensities so that individuals with a clinically significant hearing loss can be identified quickly in a large population (e.g. school children). Such audiometers are usually used outside the hospital, in schools and clinics. Those individuals who fail a screening test of hearing would usually be referred for more precise testing methods in the audiology department at the hospital or other referral centre.

Sealed source r=3

This term is applied to small containers (tubes or needles) containing radioactive material which can be inserted into tumours, or applied to the surface, to provide localized radiotherapy. The containers are typically platinum or irridium alloys, or, in the case of tubes, silver. The radioactive elements are normally radium or caesium-137. Such devices are found in the radiotherapy or oncology department.

Section (ultrasound) scanner n=3 c=5,6 r=1

This is an ultrasonic B-scanner which presents echo amplitude as brightness on the screen and relates the point of origin of the echo to the correct point on the screen of a cathode ray tube. There are many types of section scanner including static B-scanners on which the ultrasonic transducer is moved over the skin by hand, its position and orientation being related to the cathode ray display by a set of potentiometers mounted on an articulated connecting arm between the transducer and the scanner. In the case of moving picture scanners the orientation and position of the transducer, or active element on a multi-element transducer, is related to the display by a complex electronic mechanism.

The section scan takes the form of a 'bacon slice' of the tissue immediately beneath the scanning plane. See also B-scanner, Real-time ultrasonic scanner, Linear array scanner and Phased array scanner.

Semi-closed circuit r=2

During anaesthesia gases are delivered to the patient through the breathing circuit such that exhaled gases may be completely discharged from the circuit, or they may be wholly or partially rebreathed. A semi-closed circuit is one in which they are partially re-inhaled, intentionally or otherwise. The most common breathing circuit (the Magill or Mapleson A) is such a circuit in which a carbon dioxide absorber may be included or not.

Sensitometer n=1 c=2 r=7

A sensitometer is a device for imprinting an image on a photographic or X-ray film in known steps of exposure. The object is to provide a standard set of exposures, usually in the form of a staircase pattern which can be read by a densitometer after the film is processed.

In practice the film is placed in the sensitometer and a standard amount of light is emitted through a mask which includes a step wedge. Such devices are used in photographic laboratories, but in medical use their application is for assurance of X-ray film quality and film processor performance.

Shaker n=20 c=1,2

This is a relatively simple device which causes a long rod to oscillate, and attached to this rod are several clamps which hold test tubes or small flasks in which chemical reactions are taking place. The shaking action causes mixing of the contents of the flasks or tubes ensuring a uniform chemical reaction. Shakers are used in the clinical chemistry laboratory where long periods of agitation are required.

Short-wave diathermy apparatus n=4 c=4 r=3,10

Internal heating (diathermy) can be caused by including a part of the body in a strong electromagnetic field of short wavelength. In the physiotherapy department short-wave generators are used to heat parts of the body which are injured, stiff, painful, or inflamed. The affected part (e.g. knee or shoulder) is placed between two insulated metal plates to which the short-wave oscillator is connected. Heating occurs because of dielectric losses in the body tissues and fluids. A common frequency is 27 MHz.

The electromagnetic field may also be applied using an insulated wire wound around the area being treated, or wound into a flat or spiral coil (a 'pancake coil') which is placed close to the skin. There are various treatment regimes involving continuous, pulsed and pulsing waveforms.

Siegles speculum

This is a speculum attached to a pneumatic tube and hand bellows used to momentarily raise the pressure in the external ear in order to observe the mobility or distension of the eardrum. It may be self contained or designed as an attachment for an otoscope.

Sigmoidoscope n=5 c=3,4 r=4

Direct viewing, treatment, or biopsy sampling, may be achieved using an illuminated hollow tube passed into the rectum and sigmoid colon. Nowadays a flexible colonoscope would normally be used employing optic fibres to convey the light and to return the image to the eyepiece. In this case the device would have more general application for viewing the colon well beyond the ascending section.

Single-needle device

A few years ago haemodialysis was usually performed by connecting the haemodialysis machine to an arteriovenous shunt by which two plastic tubes passed through the skin at the wrist or lower leg, one into an artery, and the other into a vein. After dialysis these tubes were connected together forming a shunt between artery and vein. More recently an arteriovenous fistula has been used by which an artery and a vein are surgically joined internally to form a bulb of blood at the joint. During haemodialysis two needles are passed into the bulb (fistula), one for withdrawing blood and the other for returning it.

The procedure can be performed using a single needle through which blood is first withdrawn, fed to the dialyser, and then returned. This procedure requires a single-needle device which times the withdrawal procedure and return period, and clamps the tubes to the dialyser in turn to enable the use of a single line to the patient. With earlier haemodialysis machines this has required an external device but modern machines incorporate this into the main console.

Skin resistance meter n=1 c=2

The galvanic resistance of the skin is sometimes measured to demonstrate changes in mental activity such as surprise, pain, strain, and uneasiness, often with metal electrodes placed on the palm and wrist. The resistance is measured by including the resistance between the electrodes in the arms of a bridge circuit which can be balanced to give a null reading on a meter. The bridge is normally energized by a small direct current. The device is sometimes known as a lie detector.

Slit lamp n=1 c=4

This device is used in ophthalmology for tonometry (measurement of pressure within the eye), and measurement of corneal thickness and anterior chamber depth. The instrument provides a narrow slit of light which is projected into the eye, and reflections from this are detected obliquely with a travelling microscope to measure the position of the reflecting surfaces. It may also be used during contact lens fitting.

Smart Bristow faradic coil r=10

Pulses of electric current as used in faradic treatment in physiotherapy departments are usually generated by electronic apparatus with facilities for pulsating the bursts of electric pulses. In older machines a faraday coil is used which generates the pulses by the interruption of current to an inductor (similar to a car ignition coil). The Smart Bristow faradic coil used in physiotherapy apparatus has a retractable iron core which is moved in and out of the coil to change the strength of the pulses.

Sona-graph n=1 c=5

This is an audio-spectrum analyser which presents a display on a cathode ray tube showing time in the X-direction, frequency in the Y-direction and amplitude proportional to the density (brightness) of the picture. As the CRT spot moves in the Y-direction the centre frequency of the analysing band pass filter increases. Such devices would be used in the speech therapy department to assist in the understanding of abnormal speech patterns. This is also called a spectrograph.

Sound level meter n=3 c=2,4 r=3,8

A basic sound level meter consists of a microphone, an amplifier, rectifier and logarithmic scale meter calibrated in decibels above a reference level. Sometimes called (correctly) a sound pressure level meter it is used to measure sound level in rooms, levels of speech and (when coupled to an artificial ear or artificial mastoid) for calibrating audiometers . It may be used for environmental sound measurements such as in audiometric booths or in the audiology department for adjusting one's voice level during simple speech perception tests, or for testing the performance of apparatus.

More complex versions may include true r.m.s. averaging, variable time constant averaging of sound, peak sound level recording, and also filters or weighting networks. Filters may be used to measure the sound level in particular frequency bands as a method of analysing the frequency content of environmental sound or for measuring distortion of pure tones from the harmonic spectrum. The filters are often arranged in octaves or part octaves for this purpose.

Weighting networks may be used instead of filters to modify the frequency response of the amplifier so as to provide a reading which more closely approximates to the perceived loudness of sounds. The most commonly used weighting is the A-weighting, calibrated in dBA which is suitable for relatively quiet sound levels (about 40 dBSPL at 1 kHz). For higher sound levels the dBB and dBC scales are more appropriate. Other weighting characteristics are used for specific sounds such as jet aircraft noise. Without filters or weighting networks the meter is said to be in the linear mode, in which case the sounds are expressed in decibels above a standard level (dBSPL) of 0.00002 Pa, which corresponds to an average for the normal hearing threshold at 1 kHz.

Spectrascribe $n=1$ $c=4$

This provides a real-time analysis of speech patterns displaying frequency, amplitude and time on a storage oscilloscope. A print-out may be obtained on ultraviolet sensitive paper. This is similar to the sona-graph, or audio-spectrum analyser and may be found in the speech therapy department.

Spectrograph/spectroscope $r=1$

This is a general term used for electronic devices which analyse signals into a histogram-type display of two of the features of the signals.

An example is an audio-spectrum analyser which shows the relative intensities of the various frequency bands in a speech waveform. These can be used to assist a patient with speech difficulties to form the sounds properly. Another version of the same type of instrument might be used to display or record frequency distribution of the doppler-shifted components scattered from the blood as detected by an ultrasonic blood velocity meter.

Spectroscopes are also used to display the energy distribution of radioactive decay as a histogram of the number of counts in each of many energy bands. These might also be called pulse-height analysers. The particular reactions involved may be identified from the energy spectrum.

Spectrophotometer n=5 c=4,5 r=9

This is a general term for a class of instruments of which photometers and colorimeters are examples. Spectrophotometry is based on the property of some substances of clinical interest to absorb or emit radiation at character-istic wavelengths. In laboratory applications, the wavelengths involved are ultraviolet (200–400 nm) or infrared (700–800 nm), but the majority are in the visible range (400–700 nm). The spectrophotometer usually has four main components: a light source, a wavelength selector (a filter, prism, or diffraction grating), a sample chamber (cuvette), and a detector and readout device.

The light source may be a hydrogen or deuterium discharge lamp for ultraviolet, or a tungsten filament lamp for other wavelengths. The filter selects a specific range of wavelengths for transmission to the cuvette or detector and may be a special glass or interference filter with layers of dielectric with high and low refractive indices or it may use a prism or diffraction grating as a monochromator from which individual wavelengths with very narrow bandwidths can be selected by rotating the angle between the light source and the detector. The cuvette is usually a special glass or plastic chamber. The detector (photometer) may be a photomultiplier tube or semiconductor device.

Flame photometers also exist in which the sample is ionized in a gas flame to emit light or to absorb it by using the flame in place of the cuvette. Flame photometers determine the concentrations of pure metals. The absorption type of flame photometer is sometimes called an atomic absorption spectrophotometer.

In a colorimeter the particular chemical is identified after mixing with a specific reagent to produce a material with a characteristic colour or wavelength for easier identification in the spectrophotometer. Since only a single colour is to be detected these normally use filters rather than monochromators.

Spectrophotometers are found in the clinical chemistry department for the chemical analysis of samples taken from blood, urine, the tissues, and other body fluids.

Speech amplifier n=2 c=1,2

Patients with quiet voices, typically after laryngectomy or with Parkinson's disease, may use a pocket-sized speech amplifier with a hand-held or boom-mounted microphone. Such devices are used by the speech therapy department.

Speech audiometer n=2 c=3 r=3

An excellent, though rather subjective measure of the extent of a hearing defect can be obtained by the delivery of speech (usually lists or groups of words or sentences) at a known sound pressure level and scoring the number of words correctly recognized. The speech is normally generated from a tape recording of the word lists played through an audiometer so that the sound level delivered can be changed to known levels for each part of the test. Clearly the level of co-operation of the patient is crucial to the correct interpretation of the results. Speech audiometers would be found in the audiology department.

Speech synthesizer n=2 c=2,3

There are now many integrated electronic circuits available at relatively low cost for the production of words or part words (phonyms). These can be made use of by people with speech difficulties. Entry may be via a keyboard or some other device appropriate to the disability of the patient. It is expected that such devices will increase in popularity as the technology develops.

Speech trainer n=5 c=1

Individuals who are profoundly deaf from an early age often have great difficulty in developing normal speech because they do not hear their own voices well. In assisting them to develop speech an amplifying device is often used to feed back their own speech via headphones at a greatly amplified level. The device itself consists of a microphone, an amplifier with variable output and a pair of headphones. The same device is sometimes used as a communication aid for the deaf.

Such devices would usually be found in the speech therapy department or in schools for the deaf.

Sphygmomanometer n=300 c=1 r=3

This is the commonest form of blood pressure measuring apparatus used in every ward, theatre and clinic of the hospital. The measurement is indirect (i.e. there is no sensor inside the body) and is subjective, and therefore can result in large errors, particularly if the operator is inexperienced. The pressure is usually measured by a mercury-in-glass manometer but an aneroid gauge is sometimes used.

A rubber bag is attached to the upper arm under a cuff which is wrapped around the arm and secured by Velcro tape. The bag is connected by tubing to the manometer and to an inflating device in the form of a bulb. The bag is inflated by squeezing the bulb until the pressure exceeds the arterial pressure. This condition is detected by a stethoscope placed over the brachial artery just below the elbow since no sound is heard from the closed artery. A valve adjacent to the bulb is then partially opened so that the bag deflates slowly. Sounds from the artery are first heard when the applied pressure just fails to occlude the artery at the peak of the arterial pressure cycle (the systolic pressure). This pressure is noted and the applied pressure allowed to continue falling until the artery fails to occlude even at the lowest point of the arterial pressure cycle (the diastolic pressure). This point is identified from characteristic sounds (the Korotkoff sounds) at this point, which the operator learns to recognize. The two pressures, systolic and diastolic, are recorded as the patient's blood pressure and are typically around 120 and 80 mmHg respectively.

Automatic indirect blood pressure recording devices exist which operate the pressurizing and depressurizing cycle and which detect the systolic and diastolic pressures from pulsations in the cuff pressure, sounds detected by a microphone under the cuff or from the arterial movements as detected by an ultrasonic doppler transducer under the cuff. Such devices have proved useful when the patient is immobile (in intensive care and under anaesthesia) but may be subject to patient movement artefacts in other situations.

Spinning top n=1 c=1 r=7

This is a very simple device for checking the exposure timer on a diagnostic X-ray set. It consists of a round lead disc, 10 cm or so in diameter with holes (e.g. seven of 3 mm diameter) drilled at various distances from the centre. The disc has a knob at the centre with which it can be set spinning by hand upon its solid base.

The output from an X-ray set is pulsating at the mains supply frequency (50 or 60 Hz), or at twice or six times this frequency depending on the rectification method employed in the set. The spinning top is placed over an X-ray film cassette and an exposure made while the disc is rotating, thus imprinting a series of dots on the film showing the number of pulses delivered during the exposure. For instance, for half-wave rectification at 50 Hz, ten dots would indicate an exposure time of 0.2 second.

Only one hole is uncovered at a time (the others being plugged) so that a number of time checks can be conducted using the same film.

Spirometer/spirograph n=3 c=2 r=2,6

These measure the volumes of gases breathed in or out. They are usually displacement (bell) devices, a bellows, or a small turbine device with gears to drive a pointer. The displacement type consists of an inverted closed cylinder with its open end immersed in water. The expired gases are fed into the cylinder through a tube opening just above the water level inside the cylinder. As more gas is fed in, the cylinder must rise. The cylinder is usually linked to a pen which writes on a rotating drum (kymograph). Thus respiratory gas volume movements can be recorded on a graph against time.

Such devices are used in lung-function studies in the respiratory laboratory, and they may also be used by anaesthetists and cardiologists. An alternative method of spirometry is to replace the cylinder and water by a large soft bellows, one side of which is coupled to a pen.

In the lung-function laboratory it is used routinely to measure the vital capacity (VC) and the forced expiratory volume (FEV). The vital capacity is simply the volume which can be breathed out after maximum inspiration and the FEV1 is the volume which can be breathed out in 1 second. For accurate records a correction must be made to take account of the different temperature of the gas in the lungs and in the spirometer. Special tables are available to make this correction. Spirometers are also used for tests involving continuous breathing such as residual volume (RV) and transfer factor (TL) measurements, but in conjunction with other apparatus.

An anaesthetist is likely to use a spirometer to monitor the tidal volume or the minute volume of a patient connected to a lung ventilator, and so the above types would be unsuitable. He may therefore use a device which produces an electronic integration of gas velocity such as the Wright's respiration monitor, an anemometer which is calibrated in volume flow, or the ventilator may have a spirometer bellows which indicates tidal volume by the distance between the two end states. The normal ventilator bellows gives some indication of tidal volume but errors are possible due to leaks, compression of gas due to the action of the ventilator, changes in gas composition in the lungs, fresh gas flow, etc. This form of spirometry can only be conducted accurately in the expiratory part of the circuit.

Spirometers are also used in the calculation of cardiac output (litres of blood/minute) using the Fick method which requires a calculation of oxygen consumption. This is achieved using a spirometer in conjunction with a carbon dioxide absorber. The oxygen consumption is the reduction in volume/minute of the quantity of gas in the spirometer.

Ultrasonic spirometers also exist which detect gas flow from ultrasound transit time up and down the tube. Another type exists which counts vortices produced by the gas flow past baffles in the transducer.

Stat analyser $n=30$ $c=4$ $r=6$

This is a discrete sample analyser used in a chemical pathology emergency laboratory or intensive care unit when chemical analysis of a small number of samples is required. These are used when an autoanalyser is not available to perform the test, or rapid results are required. Typical measurements might be of potassium, sodium, calcium ion concentration, etc.

Step wedge n=1 c=1,2 r=7

Sometimes known as a penetrometer or penetrameter, it consists of an aluminium block or laminate of several strips of aluminium forming a staircase. It is used to test X-ray sets (and film processors). It is placed on the film or cassette such that the increasing thickness of each step of the wedge causes different amounts of X-ray absorption so that the film is exposed to a different extent under each step of the wedge. The step wedge is placed over different portions of the film as X-rays of different kilovoltage (kV) and milliampere-seconds (mAs) are delivered. Any marked differences or irregularities in strip density indicate malfunction of the X-ray set or processor.

Special X-ray test cassettes exist which include copper step wedges and are used for calculations of the kV_p of X-ray beams.

The print on the X-ray film created by exposure under a step wedge is also called a step wedge, even if created by a sensitometer, or simulated on a video screen.

Sterilizer n=20 c=1,3,4 r=2

Sterilization of instruments and equipment may be effected by several methods according to the durability of the item and the degree of sterilization required. Methods include the following:

1. Dry heat. Some items may be sterilized by heating to 150°C or more in a special oven. The items are normally wrapped in special paper sealed with tape which includes a colour indicator to show when the process has been completed. Some care is required to ensure that items made of different materials are not damaged due to the differential expansion rates of the components.
2. Pasteurization. Delicate items (e.g. some plastic items) may be sterilized by heating in water to 70-75°C for a minimum of 20 minutes. Most infective agents are destroyed but the process is only really suitable where a high degree of sterilization is not required.
3. Boiling. Boiling for a least 10 minutes is a satisfactory method for most metal items. Tubing and instruments with complex contours may not be adequately sterilized.
4. Autoclaving. This is probably the most satisfactory and widely used method. Instruments are packed in special paper sealed with an indicator tape to show completion of the process, and are placed in a pressure

vessel which first exhausts the air before releasing high-pressure (and therefore high-temperature) steam into the chamber. Because of the vacuum created initially, the steam penetrates to every part of the equipment. After a few minutes (depending on the steam temperature used) the steam is evacuated leaving the instruments dry. Many plastic items and some rubbers are damaged by repeated autoclaving.

5. Chemical sterilization. Fumigation or immersion in anti-bacterial agents may be appropriate for some items. However this cannot provide reliable sterilization with complex items, or tubing unless great care is taken. An exception is ethylene oxide sterilization which employs a process similar to the autoclaving cycle to ensure total penetration of all contours. Such machines are complex and expensive to purchase and operate, and require meticulous anti-pollution measures since the gas is highly toxic.

6. Gamma rays. Many disposable items are sterilized by irradiation from a gamma-ray source. This is highly effective but disrupts the polymer structure of some plastics causing hardening, decomposition and discolouring.

Sterotoner n=0 r=4

Substitution of audible signals for printed characters as an aid for the blind has its origins well before modern computers. This device is the trade name for a converter which produces characteristic sounds for each letter read by a special detector head. With training, reading could be accomplished at 40-60 words per minute. This particular apparatus is no longer available, but the general principle may be re-used in other apparatus.

Stethoscope r=9

Sounds from the heart, chest and peripheral circulation, which were originally detected by pressing an ear to the skin, are now detected using a stethoscope. This is normally a small bell-shaped end-piece pressed on to the skin and coupled to a flexible tube, splitting to feed two ear-pieces. The performance of this system is roughly equivalent to that achieved by direct application of the ear, with some amplification provided by standing waves within the system. Sound levels detected and the frequency response depend upon the pressure applied to the skin (low frequencies are lost by higher pressure) and by how well the ear-pieces fit into the ears.

The diagnostic accuracy achieved using a stethoscope depends to a large extent on the experience and skill of the clinician, since it is very hard to give a verbal description of the sounds. Electronic types exist to amplify and modify the sounds but these have not been generally accepted by clinicians, partly because the sounds generated are unfamiliar to them.

Stethoscopes also exist which detect the heart sounds from within the oesophagus. Ultrasonic foetal heart detectors are also sometimes (incorrectly) call stethoscopes.

Stimulator r=3

This loose term is usually taken to mean an electrical stimulator for inducing muscle contraction during anaesthesia, physiotherapy, or during diagnostic procedures. It can of course apply to photostimulators, used during electroretinography, auditory stimulators used during electric response audiometry, or chemical stimulators (stimulants) used in therapy. More details can be found under the specific headings.

Stirrer n=20 c=1

This is a relatively simple device used for stirring the contents of small flasks to ensure good mixing during slow chemical reactions. The usual form of the device is a small box on which the flask is placed. Inside the box is a motor rotating a small magnet just beneath the top surface of the box. Another small magnet encapsulated in a plastic coating is dropped into the flask and this rotates in sympathy with the magnet rotating beneath. This causes continual stirring of the contents of the flask.

Stomach pump n=1 c=3,4

Stomach washout may be achieved by the simple procedure of passing a tube into the stomach and pouring in fluid through a funnel, and then lowering the tube to siphon out the contents. Automated versions exist which provide a washing cycle, and such devices may also be adapted for investigation purposes in which samples of stomach contents are removed at intervals into vials for examination.

Stop-action (ultrasonic) scanner r=1

Stop-action scanning may be used to provide a frozen ultrasonic B-scan corresponding to a particular time in the cardiac cycle to identify the positions of the valve leaflets. It can be applied to a hand-operated static B-scanner by using the ECG R-wave to trigger the mechanism so that the image contains only lines corresponding to a particular time. Thus images of 'valves open' or 'valves closed' positions may be built up.

The same principle may be employed with a real-time scanner in which the frame freeze facility is invoked at the desired time in the cardiac cycle.

Storage cathode ray tube n=3 c=3 r=3

A graph, or a complete picture can be built up on a special CRT screen which retains the image as electrostatic charge on a fine insulating mesh behind the screen. When the whole screen is illuminated by low-velocity electrons from a 'flood gun' the electrostatic mesh forms a mask so that the original image can be seen on the screen.

These CRTs have been used extensively in electronic test instruments and in ultrasonic B-scanners because of the ease with which the image can be stored and erased. The main drawback (for B-scanning at least) is that the display is bi-stable, so that each point on the screen is either blank or at maximum brightness. This is only suitable for line drawing since no 'grey scale' is possible. Many bi-stable CRTs can also be driven in 'variable persistence' mode which does allow some modulation of the brightness, but the image is continually fading. The variable persistence facility is useful during the setting-up procedure for some tests.

It is expected that high-speed computer graphics memories, in conjunction with conventional short-persistence CRTs or TV-type monitors, will supplant storage CRTs.

Strain gauge transducer n=40 r=2,9

These measure strain (stretch) and produce an electrical signal, usually by changing electrical resistance as the strain increases. They are used in some pressure transducers to measure the bending of the diaphragm and are also used in force transducers and displacement transducers. The strain gauge element is often a thin metallic film or wire which is glued on to the part which is being stretched.

An excellent list of strain gauge transducer materials and performance is given on page 52 of reference 9.

Suction catheter r=2

The suction catheter or nozzle is the terminal piece for a suction machine or unit which is used to draw up blood, mucus or vomit from operation sites or the airways. These are often transparent or have a transparent section so that the aspirated material can be seen passing up the tube to the reservoir. Often the nozzle section has a hole in the side which reduces the suction pressure (i.e. provides less vacuum) at the end of the nozzle, but allows the suction to be raised to a maximum simply by placing a finger over the end. They are often tapered at the end, allowing the main length of the catheter to be wider in diameter to prevent obstruction as debris passes along it.

Suction electrode r=9

In electrocardiography, the precordial (chest) electrode may sometimes consist of a short metal cylinder which makes contact with the skin at its base, which is smeared with conductive electrode jelly. The upper end of the tube is connected to a rubber bulb which is squeezed and then released as the tube makes contact with the skin. It adheres to the skin by suction while the recording is made and then it can be moved to another site. The contact impedance is higher than for the larger surface area electrodes used for the limb leads.

Suction machine n=100 c=3,4 r=2

This usually refers to a portable suction apparatus used in wards and theatres for aspirating fluids and vomit from the mouth and airways, and from operation sites by sucking the material through a catheter into a bottle. The term could also apply to devices which operate from piped vacuum supplies or bottle gas cylinders but is more commonly used to mean electric suction units which contain a vacuum pump (piston, diaphragm, or rotary vane), bacterial filter, vacuum gauge, trap for moisture (or any debris accidentally drawn into the mechanism), a reservoir for the aspirated material, and a suction catheter or nozzle. They may be intended to provide high or low vacuum, and high and low flow rates. Low vacuum is used for post-operative wound drainage.

The main reservoir is usually a glass bottle with volume marks up the side and sometimes this has a float valve so that the vacuum is cut off before the bottle becomes full enough to allow the contents to be drawn into the pipework of the pumping mechanism. However, frothing of the contents can sometimes defeat the float valve mechanism.

They may sometimes be described as high-grade or low-grade suction machines, which relates to the degree of vacuum achieved. High-grade suction machines are used for rapid aspiration of fluids and debris (such as vomit), whereas low-grade machines are used for post-operative wound drainage.

Suction therapy apparatus n=1 c=3

Equipment exists for use in the physiotherapy department which can provide pulsating suction to flexible cups applied to the skin. The suction is often used to retain electrodes on the skin which are being used for some form of electrical therapy (e.g. interferential therapy). However, a therapeutic effect is claimed for the 'suction massage' itself.

The suction apparatus may have up to four outlets to which suction cups may be connected and there may be controls to set the strength of suction and the rate and duration of the pulsations.

Superficial X-ray treatment unit n=1 c=5,6 r=3

These are medium-energy (50–150 kV) X-ray machines with suitable collimators and applicators for treating surface cancers.

These are found in radiotherapy departments and in some skin clinics.

Surgical diathermy machine n=15 c=4 r=2

Localized heating of tissue without muscle twitch or spasm can be effected by passing a large alternating current of high frequency through parts of the body. This is surgical diathermy or electrosurgery. If the power is sufficient, the temperature reached causes coagulation of the blood or even disintegration of the tissue due to boiling.

This technique is employed in a controlled manner during surgery to seal small blood vessels by coagulation, and to cut through layers of tissue. Cutting and coagulation is achieved by applying electric current to the tissues via small hand-held probes (electrodes). The current flows out of the body (usually) through a very large electrode placed on the skin at some remote site (e.g. on the thigh). At this electrode (the indifferent electrode) the current density is very low, so little heating occurs. However, at the hand-held electrode the density is very high due to its small contact area, and so great heat is developed.

Diathermy currents may be generated by valve or transistor circuits and may include a range of protection and monitoring systems. The frequencies used are typically in the range 0.5 to 3 MHz and so it is difficult to achieve true earth-free operation due to the capacitance between the patient and earth, and the capacitance of the leads of monitoring equipment. Most versions have power output up to a few hundred watts, with slightly higher power necessary for urology applications where the surgery often takes place under water (in the bladder). Low power versions exist, sometimes called hyfrecators, for excision of warts, polyps, and skin flaps.

The system described above is monopolar, whereas bipolar systems are available in which the heating currents only flow between the two tips of special forceps. These are useful for fine work and when the patient has a pacemaker which might malfunction in the presence of the very large circulating high-frequency current.

Swan-Ganz catheter r=4

The pressure in the left atrium of the heart may be estimated by measuring the pulmonary wedge pressure. This technique uses an inflated balloon-tipped catheter, which is passed through the chambers of the heart from an incision in a peripheral artery. The catheter is directed by the force of the blood flow on the balloon. It is eventually positioned so that the tip of the catheter is wedged into one of the small vessels leading to the lungs. Since this blocks the local flow, the pressure in the capillary bed of the lungs can be measured. The pressure across the capillary bed of the lungs is small and so this approximates to the left atrial pressure.

Such catheters can be positioned without fluoroscopic (X-ray) assistance and can be used for medium-term monitoring in the intensive care unit as well as in the cardiac catheter laboratory.

The left atrial pressure is a useful index of cardiac performance.

Syringe pump n=50 c=2 r=4

A motorized syringe is often used to maintain a constant slow infusion of a drug. These normally take standard disposable syringes on a rack which is driven by a worm drive coupled to a gearbox and motor, or directly to a stepping motor. These usually work from the mains electricity supply but may also be battery operated or clockwork. The battery and clockwork types can usually be made small enough to be carried by the patient in a special pocket or holster, in cases where slow infusion is required over a long period.

Some machines have two syringes mounted on them so that one is filling while the other is discharging, and there is a valve arrangement to allow changeover. Although these are relatively simple devices, they may be unsuitable for some tasks because of unsatisfactory drive compliance, jerking of the syringe as the plunger is pressed, or applying excessive pressures when there is a blockage. Some types lack adequate alarm circuits.

T

T-piece circuit r=2

Gas anaesthesia is normally applied via a breathing circuit which includes an expiratory valve. This releases excess gas (mainly during exhalation) via a pressure relief valve. One adverse effect of this is to offer some resistance to exhalation. In paediatric anaesthesia this problem can be avoided by using a T-piece circuit (Mapleson classification type E) in which the fresh gas feed is connected to a T-piece which connects on one side to the patient (by a mask or endotracheal tube) and on the other to a length of corrugated breathing tube. Fresh gas fills the tube during the expiratory pause and this is taken in during inspiration. During expiration the waste gases pass out down the tube. Obviously there is some rebreathing but this is limited by the flow rate of fresh gas.

An important modification of this circuit is the inclusion of a double-ended reservoir bag at the end of the length of breathing tube. The distal end of this bag can be occluded with a finger during the inspiratory phase of assisted ventilation and release during the rest of the cycle. This is the Rees T-piece circuit.

Tape recorder n=20 c=1,2 r=3

These store information by magnetizing small particles on the surface of a plastic tape on open reels, on reels in cassettes or cartridges, or the same principle may be applied on discs, drums or strips (e.g. magnetic credit cards). There are several types of tape recorder:

1. Direct recorders (DR). The tape is drawn past a metal or ferrite ring which has a small gap in it at its point of contact with the tape. The ring is subjected to a varying magnetic flux (the signal) by a coil wound round it so that the tape is magnetized to an extent corresponding to the signal amplitude. On replay the tape passes the same head (usually) and induces current in the coil corresponding to the extent of tape magnetization. Unfortunately the current induced depends on the rate of change of magnetism passing the head and so slow changes are lost, and also very rapid changes are lost due to different effects connected with the width of the head gap and the tape speed. Thus direct recording machines are only

suitable for a limited range (e.g. the audible frequencies). This frequency range can be extended by rotating the tape head at high speed using the method employed in video recorders.

2. FM (frequency modulated) recorders. The recording of low frequencies and steady signals can be achieved by representing the voltage to be recorded as the frequency of a tone which is recorded in the normal way on a direct recording machine. On playback the tone is converted back into voltage, the higher the frequency the higher the voltage. Such recorders are useful for logging relatively slow-moving signals such as physiological pressures. The frequency response of FM recorders depends on the tape speed and width of the head gap. A steady tape speed is essential since this affects the frequency of the tone when replayed.

3. Digital recorders. Signals may be recorded by representing the signal as a series of numbers in binary code on the tape. Such recording is relatively independent of variations in tape speed and the principle is used extensively in computers.

4. Video recorders. These are direct recording machines with very high bandwidth sufficient to register television signals (approximately 5 MHz). There are several methods in use (e.g. Umatic, VHS, Betamax) which are mutually incompatible.

TcpO₂ monitor

Transcutaneous partial oxygen pressure monitor, see Transcutaneous oxygen monitor.

Teleisotope unit n=1 c=6 r=3

High-activity radionuclides such as caesium-137 and cobalt-60 can be used to provide high-energy gamma-ray beams for the treatment of tumours. A teleisotope unit delivers the beam from outside the body, passing through the skin to the site to be treated.

Cobalt-60 is the most commonly used gamma-ray source for this form of teletherapy since it is highly active, and has a long half-life (5.5 years) and produces radiation at 1.17 and 1.33 MeV. The cobalt source contains a number of cobalt-60 discs in a double stainless steel container with screwed and brazed lids. The source is contained within a treatment head which may weigh one ton. The head may include all of the shielding, and the mechanism for rotating the source or collimator to expose or hide the source itself.

The radiation is delivered to the patient via a set of collimators to contain the beam to the correct shape required for the treatment. The head itself may also be manipulated to deliver the beam from a number of different angles so that maximum irradiation occurs at the centre of this rotation, other parts of the body receiving proportionately less.

Such machines are found in the radiotherapy department.

Telemetry r=6,9

This literally means the measurement or recording of signals at a distance. In medical work the best known use of telemetry is in the radio transmission of ECG signals to remove the need for connecting wires to the patient. The principle has been applied experimentally to almost every other physiological variable which can be measured. Of particular interest at present is the use of radio-telemetry for monitoring the foetus during labour, allowing the mother to be freed from the constraints of a wired system. Less used techniques include implanted radio transmitters, and radio pills which are swallowed.

Strictly, telemetry refers to other forms of remote recording and examples which exist are ECG, or pacemaker performance monitoring over the telephone.

For radio telemetry each country has regulations relating to the allowable frequency, power, and modulations systems permissible for medical work.

Teletherapy apparatus n=3 c=6,7 r=3

This is a cancer treatment machine employing high-energy electromagnetic radiation delivered from a point outside the body as opposed to sealed sources of radioactive material implanted within the body.

Machines for teletherapy include high-voltage X-ray machines, linear accelerators, high-energy isotope units and neutron generators. X-ray units for teletherapy include superficial X-ray generators (50–150 kV), orthovoltage units (150–500 kV), linear accelerators to produce electron or X-ray energies between 4 and 15 MeV, and isotope units which may produce 0.66 MeV (caesium-137) or 1.17 MeV and 1.33 MeV for cobalt-60 sources.

In the case of teleisotope units the rays cannot be directed and so they are restricted by a lead collimator. The primary collimator in the treatment head confines the beam to a broad cone covering the maximum possible area to be irradiated, and a secondary collimator or applicator further restricts this for the particular treatment regime required. If this is an applicator it is placed on the skin of the patient, thus defining the source-to-skin distance (SSD).

Theraktin tunnel bath r=10

This is a semi-cylindrical frame in which are mounted four fluorescent tubes within a reflector intended to provide even irradiation of the patient. The irradiation is normally in the UVA part of the electromagnetic spectrum (280–400 nm) and is used in the physiotherapy department for increasing the skin blood supply, relief of pain, muscle relaxation, and also in treating some skin conditions.

Therapeutic diathermy equipment n=12 c=3,4 r=4

Diathermy refers to processes which produce deep heating of the tissues. Surgical diathermy used in surgery is not really diathermy at all and should be called by its proper name, electrosurgery. True diathermy is used in physiotherapy for the treatment of strains and sprains resulting in chronic inflammation, and for the relief of pain. There are three processes used to cause diathermy.

1. Shortwave diathermy. Radio frequency energy (usually 27 MHz) is applied between two metal plates so that part of the energy is absorbed in the tissue. This causes heating throughout the limb or other area under treatment.
2. Microwave diathermy. Radio-frequency energy (usually 2450 MHz) is directed at the body from an aerial. The process is similar to microwave cooking except that the microwaves are applied from one side only. Thus most heating occurs at the skin surface and diminishes with distance into the tissue.
3. Ultrasonic diathermy. Ultrasonic energy between 1 and 3 MHz is applied directly to the skin, or with a patient in a bath, relying on the absorption of ultrasound in tissue. Using intensity levels of between 1 and 3 W/cm^2 mild heat is generated internally which is particularly useful in the treatment of inflammation of joints and tendons.

Thermistor r=9

Thermistors are semiconductors made of ceramic materials which have a high negative temperature coefficient of resistance. They can be small in size (e.g. 0.5 mm in diameter) and have relatively large sensitivity to temperature changes (−3% to −5% change per °C), and have good long-term stability. Change of resistance is not linear with temperature but when employed in a bridge circuit good linearity can be achieved. The current through thermistors must be small to prevent electrical heating, and they are usually encapsulated in glass. Some electrical clinical thermometers use thermistors, often with a disposable sheath.

Thermistors are also used in breathing rate meters in which the device is taped to be in the airstream in the mouth (at the lips) or in the nose.

Thermocouple r=9

These work by the Seebeck effect, which is a combination of the Peltier effect by which a small voltage exists at the junction of two unlike metals, and a second effect credited to Lord Kelvin which produces a small voltage along a conductor in a temperature gradient. Both effects are proportional to the temperatures involved. The total voltage produced in a circuit including a number of thermocouples is zero as there is no temperature difference around the loop. Thus two thermocouples are normally employed. One is maintained at a reference temperature (e.g. the freezing point of water) and the other acts as the thermometer.

The sensitivities of common thermocouples range from 6.5 to 80 $\mu V/°C$ with accuracies from 0.25% to 1%. Several thermocouples can be arranged in series to form a thermopile to increase the sensitivity. The advantages of thermocouples are their fast response (down to 1 ms), small size (down to 12 μm diameter), ease of fabrication and long-term stability. Their disadvantages are small output voltage, low sensitivity, and need for reference temperature. Small thermocouples can be inserted into catheters and hypodermic needles. Some clinical electronic thermometers employ thermocouples.

Thermodilution cardiac output computer n=1 c=4 r=3,6

Just as cardiac output can be estimated during cardiac catheterization by means of a dye dilution computer, the dilution of a bolus of saline at a different temperature from the blood may be used to produce the same result. A fine catheter is passed up into the heart through a vein. The tip of the catheter passes through the heart into the pulmonary artery where a thermistor mounted on the catheter senses the temperature. An opening in the catheter then lies in or near to the right atrium and a bolus (e.g. 5 ml) of saline is injected rapidly through this. It mixes with the blood in the heart and temporarily depresses the temperature in the right atrium. The cardiac output (in litres/minute) can be calculated from the area under the curve of temperature depression and a knowledge of the quantity and temperature of the saline.

This technique has an advantage over dye dilution methods since it can be repeated frequently to produce information about the changes in cardiac output which may occur during treatment. Such apparatus may be found in the intensive care department and in the cardiac catheter laboratory.

In addition to the special catheter (often a Swan-Ganz catheter), which may be intended for single use, the apparatus must include a thermistor amplifier and linearizer, and a small computer. ·

Thermograph

Some disorders such as breast cancer or soft tissue injuries cause local heating of the tissues, and areas of raised temperature may be detected at the surface by a variety of methods. Apart from direct-contact thermometers there are two main alternatives. One (the thermograph or heat camera) involves the remote detection of infrared radiation enabling the construction of a map of surface temperature, and the other employs liquid crystal technology to provide a colour map of temperature. This latter may involve the spraying or painting of the skin with materials which display temperature as different colour bands, or by bringing the skin surface into contact with a special flexible screen coated with liquid crystal materials which can be viewed optically or photographically from the other side. See also Radiation thermometer and Heat camera.

Thermoluminescent dosimetry apparatus n=1 c=5 r=3

This permits an alternative to film badges for the monitoring of cumulative radiation dose to a worker exposed to ionizing radiation. Many crystalline materials can absorb ionizing radiation and store a fraction of the energy by trapping electrons at impurity atoms. If the crystal is heated, this stored energy is released and the resulting radiation is in the visible spectrum. The technique is used for assessing the age of pottery (which contains some quartz) by the energy released on heating due to the cumulative radiation dose since it was fired. In hospitals the process can be simulated by the inclusion of a small quantity of lithium fluoride in (say) Teflon (PTFE) discs. The accumulated radiation dose acquired in the working environment can be assessed by heating the disc to (say) 500°C in contact with a photomultiplier tube. This method could potentially replace conventional film badge monitoring techniques.

Thermometer r=6,9

There are four main types available:

1. Those which rely on the expansion of a liquid or solid as the temperature rises. The best known of these are the mercury-in-glass type, of which there are many variations, notably the maximum reading clinical thermometer.
2. Chemical thermometers which indicate temperature by change of state or colour. Liquid crystal material can be fabricated to change state (and optical properties) at a particular temperature. If combined with a dye the colour of the material will indicate whether temperature is above or

below the transition temperature. An array of spots of such material may be arranged to form a graduated thermometer. Such devices are available for clinical use, as are special paints for the skin which produce a colour temperature map of parts of the body.

3. Electrical thermometers. These have the advantage that the temperature sensing element can be very small (e.g. 0.5 mm) and remote from the indicating part of the instrument, or even placed inside a hypodermic needle. Electrical thermometers may use thermocouples which produce a voltage proportional to the temperature difference between two bi-metal junctions by the Seebeck effect, or they may use thermistor types which sense the change in resistance due to temperature rise which occurs in some materials.

4. Radiation thermometers. There is a known relationship between the surface temperature of an object and its radiant power. Thus temperature can be sensed remotely by detecting the infrared radiation, provided the surface in question approximates to a black body radiator. Human skin meets this requirement. Radiation thermometry is employed in thermography to produce maps of the surface temperature of parts of the human body.

Time compression analyser $r=1$

Frequency analysis of ultrasonic doppler blood flow signals can be achieved using a bank of electronic filters, but a more modern method is to use a computer to perform fast Fourier transform (FFT) analysis. Doppler blood flow signals may contain frequency components from (say) 200 Hz to 15 kHz. This wide range of frequencies cannot be analysed quickly enough in a sequential mode.

This problem is solved by dividing the signal into short periods (e.g. 10 ms) and reading these into a computer memory. These are then read out at a much faster rate (e.g. 250 times faster) and rapid analysis applied to the time compressed signal. The flow pattern is then displayed on a strip chart usually produced on a fibre-optic recorder with the frequency components (velocity components) displayed across the strip. By using the amplitude of these components as well as the frequency, the rate of blood flow may also be calculated.

Such devices may be used by vascular surgeons in the investigation of flow patterns in diseased arteries.

Time–motion (TM) scanner $n=2$ $c=5,6$ $r=1$

This is a special ultrasonic scanner used for tracing the motion of structures within the body, particularly the walls and valves of the heart. It is commonly called an M-mode (motion) scanner or an echocardiograph. In effect it is a single line B-scanner presenting the echoes immediately beneath the ultrasonic transducer and moving this line slowly across a cathode ray tube screen so that static structures draw straight lines whereas moving structures have characteristic movement patterns. For further details see M-mode scanner.

Tinnitus masker c=1,2

Tinnitus is a buzzing, whistling or ringing noise which frequently accompanies deafness. It may appear to come from one or both ears or be heard within the head. It is a very poorly understood phenomenon and very little can be done to help the tinnitus sufferer. Everyday background noises can usually cover up (mask) a patient's tinnitus and so the effect is most noticeable and distressing at quiet times of the day and especially at night. Although tinnitus is sometimes present in the absence of any hearing problems, patients with a hearing loss who use a hearing aid often find that the aid amplifies even quiet environmental sounds sufficient to produce a masking effect. However, if a hearing aid is not fitted then a tinnitus masker is sometimes prescribed.

This device looks like a conventional ear-level hearing aid except that it has no microphone, and simply emits a broad band noise into the ear. Experience so far with these devices has shown that the success rate is very dependent on the amount of support and guidance given to the patient.

Tocodynamometer

This is a device for measuring the pressure within a sphere or cylinder (such as the eye, pregnant uterus, or artery) using the principle that the pressure required to flatten a section of the wall is equal to the internal pressure. A tocodynamometer employs a flat disc which is pressed on to the object until the wall becomes flat. Usually a central pressure-measuring disc is employed with an outer guard ring so that a relatively large area is flattened but pressure is only measured from the central section. A tocodynamometer is the transducer used in the external monitoring of uterine contractions during labour using a cardiotocograph. See also Applanation tonometer, and Tonometer.

Tomographic X-ray unit n=2 c=6,7 r=7

This is a special form of diagnostic X-ray set which can produce an image of a particular layer within the body. The result differs from normal X-ray images on which all layers between the tube and the film are superimposed.

Computerized tomography (CT scanning) has become possible in the last decade and uses a scanning technique employing narrow X-ray beams to assemble information on the X-ray absorption of each point within the scanning plane. An image of this absorption pattern is produced by computer (See CT scanner).

A more widely used technique causes blurring of all the structures above or below the layer under investigation by the correlated movement of any two of the tube, object (patient), and film. The most common movement is that of the tube and film with respect to the patient, who remains stationary. The tube and film are connected in such a way that they rotate about the plane to be imaged; thereby all other layers appear blurred on the image, and only interfere with the 'plane in focus' to a small extent. The tube and film may be made to undertake a number of different motions to produce the effect such as parallel linear, arcuate linear, circular, or spiral (helical) movement.

Since the exposure is usually taken over a longer period than for conventional X-ray imaging, the X-ray intensity is lower, and therefore special film and fluorescent screen combinations are used.

Tonometer r=6,9

The basic principle of a tonometer is that when a pressurized vessel is partly collapsed by an external object the circumferential stresses are removed and the internal and external pressures are equal. This approach has been used to measure intra-ocular pressure, intra-uterine pressure during pregnancy, and to a lesser extent the intraluminal pressure or pulse waveform in some arteries.

The instrument for this is an applanation tonometer which consists of a disc and outer guard-ring which flattens the wall of the sphere or cylinder and records the pressure being applied on the central disc. For the eye a non-contact type exists which identifies the pressure within the eye by flattening a small section of the cornea by a pulse of air whose force increases linearly with time. A collimated beam of light is reflected from this section of the cornea on to a detector, and the quantity of light detected is at a maximum when the test section of the cornea is flat. See also Applanation tonometer, Guard ring tocograph and Tocodynamometer.

Tourniquet n=3 c=3

A simple tourniquet is a strapping or bandage wound tightly around a limb so that it prevents blood flow. It can be used to prevent bleeding during surgery on the extremities or to prevent blood loss from a wound (for a short period).

Automatic tourniquets exist which have inflatable cuffs, similar to blood pressure cuffs applied around the upper part of each limb, and they are inflated to reduce the return of venous blood from the limbs (i.e. to a pressure of about 50 mmHg). The object may be to reduce the load on the heart, and versions exist which automatically inflate and deflate two cuffs so that venous return is only allowed from one limb at a time. A more common use of automatic tourniquets is to prevent venous blood returning to the heart in cases when local anaesthetic is being used for surgery on limbs (Bier's block technique). High doses of the anaesthetic or analgesic can be used in the limb without affecting the rest of the body. Unfortunately there have been serious accidents with these devices and the greatest possible care is required in manufacture, maintenance and use.

Automatic tourniquets may have one or two cuffs, be inflated by a pump, by hand, or from pipeline or cylinder gas sources, and usually have a cuff pressure gauge and regulator.

Tracheostomy tube $c=1$ $r=2$

This is a special catheter for direct insertion into the trachea to relieve obstructed breathing or to effect anaesthesia. It normally has provision for connection to the normal anaesthetic equipment connectors and may have an inflatable cuff to provide a seal inside the trachea for positive pressure ventilation.

Traction apparatus $n=5$ $c=3$ $r=4$

Traction is applied to the cervical or lumbar spine through harnesses fastened to the head or pelvic area. This widens the inter-vertebral spaces which relieves nerve root compression by the inter-vertebral discs. The compression of the nerve roots causes sensations of pain, burning, tingling in the neck, shoulders and arms, or in the back, buttocks, legs and feet. Traction force is determined by the patient's tolerance and is contra-indicated in some conditions. A limiting factor is the friction of the patient on the bed and therefore split beds have been developed where the lower half is free to roll independently of the upper half.

Traction may be applied as a static force by systems of weights, pulleys and springs, or in a cycling mode with period and intensity determined empirically. Electrical programmable types also exist.

Transcutaneous aortic velograph (TAV) $n=0$ $c=5$ $r=6$

This is a device to give an indication (though not a measurement) of

246

cardiac output by processing the ultrasonic doppler signals derived from the aorta from a point on the skin on the lower part of the neck. Using a 2 MHz transducer, the width of the sound beam approximately corresponds to the diameter of the aorta and the returning signals contain velocity information which may be frequency analysed and delivered to a strip chart showing the velocity patterns of the blood. The device has not found wide acceptance although variations on the theme are being developed which have great potential application for monitoring changes in cardiac output during treatment.

Transcutaneous electrical neural stimulator (TENS) n=5 c=2 r=4

About one third of patients suffering from chronic intractable pain can benefit from this type of stimulator. Electric currents are passed between large electrodes placed on the skin over a painful area. The current causes a tingling sensation and appears to affect the pain threshold. Suitable pulse rate (20–200 pulses/s), pulse width (15–1000 μs), and output voltage (0–150 V) are chosen or found empirically according to the results obtained in each individual case.

The stimulation is normally applied for three to four hours at a time and relief from pain may last for a few hours after this. Therefore each patient will find a regime of treatment which suits his lifestyle or need for relief. It has proved useful in treating chronic pain arising from herniated discs, peripheral neuropathy, injury, arthritis, and strain. It has also been found useful in the relief of acute post-operative pain.

The stimulators may be battery operated so that they can be carried by the patient. The electrodes are relatively large (e.g. 4 cm²) in order to reduce current density at the skin surface. Development of skin rash at the electrode sites is a common complication.

The mechanisms of operation, and the reasons for success or failure in individual cases are not well understood. Such devices may be used or prescribed by the neurology department.

Transducer n=100 c=2,3 r=3,9

This is a device for the conversion of one form of energy to another. In medical work the best known examples are temperature, pressure, ion concentration, force and displacement transducers. The term could be applied to any energy-converting device such as a motor or light bulb but it is usually reserved for an electrically operated measuring device or actuator.

1. Pressure transducers. The electrical versions of these usually work by allowing the pressure to bend a diaphragm in the transducer and

247

measure the bending by resistance strain gauges arranged into a bridge circuit which may be attached to the diaphragm (as in the case of most semiconductor gauges) or they may be remote from the diaphragm (unbonded) as in the case of wire or metallic film gauges. Such devices are used extensively for recording of blood pressure (via intra-arterial or intravenous cannulae), bladder pressure, etc.

2. Temperature transducers. The thermoelectric potential between two dissimilar metals (thermocouple), or the change in resistance due to temperature (thermistor) may be used to measure and record temperatures.

3. Displacement transducers. Distance moved, or position, may be measured by a potentiometer (e.g. as used to determine the position and orientation of some ultrasonic B-scan transducers) or the ratio of inductive coupling between two coils may be varied by the movement of a third coil orferrite core (LVDT). Displacement transducers may also be used as velocity or acceleration transducers with suitable electronics.

4. Ultrasonic transducers. Sound or ultrasound maybe produced by an inductive device such as the loudspeaker or magnetostrictive transducer, or be a piezoelectric element which expands or contracts according to the applied voltage. The advantage of the latter for medical applications is that they can work at high frequencies (c.g. 5 MHz) and are reciprocal in that they can convert acoustic energy into electrical signals as well as the reverse.

An excellent list of medical transducer performance requirements is given on pages 7 and 8 of reference 9.

Transfer factor analyser n=1 c=5 r=3

When a person is unable to breathe properly, oxygen does not enter the blood in sufficient quantities. The performance of different elements in the respiration mechanism may be measured separately (such as vital capacity or residual volume), but overall performance can best be described by the transfer factor which quotes the quantity of carbon monoxide which enters the blood each minute for every mmHg of partial pressure of the gas.

Carbon monoxide is used because it is readily absorbed by the haemoglobin whereas oxygen passes in both directions and would therefore be difficult to quantify. A typical procedure might be for the patient to breathe in a measured volume of gas containing known concentrations of carbon monoxide and helium. The breath is then held for ten seconds or so to allow mixing and transfer to take place. The concentrations of the two gases are then measured in the exhaled gases. The total volume of gases in the system can then be estimated from the new concentration of the helium, which enables calculation of the expected concentration of carbon monoxide if none had been transferred to the blood. The difference between this estimated concentration and the measured concentration is the quantity absorbed.

The small concentration of carbon monoxide used (less than 1% because of its high toxicity) is measured in an infrared analyser. Carbon monoxide and dioxide gases absorb infrared light at different characteristic wavelengths and so the analyser can be specific to one or other gas. The helium analyser would be the same as described for the Helium FRC analyser.

Transfer factor analysers are found in the lung function laboratory.

Transient recorder n=1 c=4 r=3

This is a device for slowing down fast signals so they can be analysed. The signal is digitized at very high speed and stored in a buffer memory (computer-type memory). When the memory is full it can be read back at a much slower speed for analysis and display. Very rapid signals such as EEG evoked responses require this type of recorder. Transient recorders require a trigger signal to start or stop the memory. This trigger may be some stimulus such as a light flash, an audible click or an electrical stimulation.

Transmission-mode (ultrasonic) scanner r=1

Just as an X-ray computerized tomography (CT) scanner can produce a map of the X-ray absorption in a tissue section, the same principle can be applied to some organs using ultrasound. The method is not widely applicable since there are few places where ultrasound can be transmitted right through the body without encountering total reflection or high attenuation in bone or air-filled spaces. However, the breasts and testes can be scanned by this method to produce a map of ultrasound absorption for the various tissues involved. It is hoped that this will lead to a new science of tissue characterization by absorption, but instruments for clinical use are not widely available.

There are problems associated with the technique related to multiple reflections and distortions of the ultrasonic beam by the complex tissue structures. There are potential applications in examining the pathology of biopsy tissue by transmission scanners (ultrasonic microscopes) using frequencies up to 500 MHz.

The apparatus consists of an ultrasonic generator, transducers placed each side of the organ being scanned, and a receiving and amplifying circuit. A scanning mechanism is also required together with a computer to assemble the image of ultrasound absorption characteristics.

Treadmill $n=1$ $c=5,6$

A treadmill consists of a wide belt on which the patient walks against the resistance to the movement of the belt. The device includes circuits to measure the work being done in moving the belt.

Patients with heart disease may undergo changes in the ECG along with blood pressure changes during exercise. Exercise may be undertaken and measured using a treadmill or a bicycle type of ergonometer. The patient exercises on the ergonometer and measurements are made of the work output, ECG, and blood pressure. The system may have alarms for specific changes in the ECG or blood pressure.

Trend recorder $n=2$ $c=4$ $r=3$

A special purpose $X–Y$ recorder or display can be used where a very large amount of information has to be summarized. Commonly a trend recorder is used to compress many hours of a recording on to a single sheet such as in ambulatory ECG recording or foetal monitoring. The recording may be of the simple trend (up or down) of a rate, or it may be a statistical presentation (e.g. histogram) of variations in each parameter (e.g. diastolic blood pressure). Such recorders are often small computers.

Tuning fork $n=50$ $c=1$ $r=8$

Tuning forks are used routinely to make a crude assessment of the extent and nature of the patient's deafness. They provide two mechanisms of transmitting sound to the ear:

1. By air conduction. This is the normal mechanism by which sound is radiated from the vibrating forks.
2. By bone conduction. The footplate of the tuning fork is pressed against the patient's forehead or mastoid bone (behind the ear). Sounds are thus transmitted as vibrations through the skull to the inner ear. Tuning forks used in hospitals therefore have a circular footplate (about 2 cm in diameter) whereas tuning forks designed for musical applications have a pointed end.

Hospital tuning forks come in a wide range of frequencies at octave intervals although the most popular are 256 and 512 Hz.

Tunnel bath $r=10$

Phototherapy, usually employing infrared light, may be applied from a radiant heat source over part of the patient to be treated in the physiotherapy department, or an array of lamps may be used in a special frame forming a tunnel over the patient or part to be treated. The main effect is superficial heating causing increased blood supply, relief of pain, muscle relaxation and perhaps biochemical effects. Similar types exist employing ultraviolet fluorescent tubes providing UVA (280–400 nm), sometimes called the Theraktin tunnel.

Turbidimeter r=5

If the substance to be examined can be made into a suspension or a finely divided colloid then the turbidity will be proportional to the concentration. If the turbidity is not too great and the particles small enough then the turbidity will relate to the amount of light absorbed in passage through it. Usually light in the red end of the spectrum will be used but the exact wavelength is not important. Such devices are sometimes used in the chemical pathology department. The construction of the instrument is broadly similar to a densitometer.

Tympanometer n=3 c=4 r=3

This is also called a middle ear impedance (or admittance) audiometer or an acoustic impedance meter, although the term is often used to describe a simple automatic machine having a restricted range of facilities. It is used to measure the sound transmission properties of the middle ear (ear drum, malleus, incus, stapes to oval window on the cochlea). It works by applying a known sound pressure to a sealed volume in the outer ear and detecting the sound level changes as the outer ear pressure is varied through a small range above and below the atmospheric pressure. Transmission through the ear drum is best when the delivered pressure is the same as the middle ear pressure (i.e. in the eustachian tube) and it falls off above and below this pressure as the ear drum stiffens as a result of the pressure differential. The resulting graph of sound transmission against pressure is plotted automatically on an X–Y recorder and is calibrated in either acoustic impedance or as effective air volume.

It is useful for demonstrating pressure in the middle ear when the eustachian tube is blocked and for showing defects in the mechanical transmission mechanism of the small middle ear bones.

Such instruments are used in the audiology department. See also Acoustic impedance meter for further information.

U

Ultrafiltration apparatus r=3

Water may be encouraged to pass through a semipermeable membrane between two fluids of roughly equal concentration by applying a pressure differential. This is similar to reverse osmosis but describes the situation when the osmotic pressure is small, and is called ultrafiltration. The technique is employed in haemodialysis to bring about a shift of water from the patient via the dialysing membrane.

The removal of large quantities of water from the patient causes a reaction which can be avoided by the correct sequencing of the two operations of ultrafiltration and haemodialysis.

A haemodialysis machine normally has the facility for adjusting the pressure between the blood and the dialysate solution across the dialysing membrane. Excessive pressures may, however, cause rupture of the membranes. Pressures up to about 400 mmHg are used.

Ultrafiltration monitor

This device monitors the movement of fluid through a dialyser membrane caused by the pressure gradient created by a positive blood pressure on one side of the membrane and a negative dialysate pressure on the other. The monitor is sometimes a separate non-intrusive device, using electronic means of measurement. On some machines the device is active and includes the ability to control fluid movement by volumetric pumps.

Ultrasonic blood flow rate meter n=3 c=2,4,5 r=9

An ultrasonic flowmeter may be used in place of an electromagnetic flowmeter to measure the instantaneous flow rate of blood. Ultrasound can be beamed through the skin, and thus measurements can be made from outside the body. Advanced types of ultrasonic flowmeters can also measure the flow profiles within blood vessels providing a potentially powerful tool for the assessment of vascular disease.

There are various methods by which blood flow can be recorded using ultrasound including transit time methods in which the blood velocity is calculated from the time taken to cross the vessel oblique to the direction of

252

flow. More commonly a continuous wave of ultrasound is transmitted through the vessel and received on a transducer adjacent to the first which picks up the back-scattered ultrasound from the blood in a zone where the transmitting and receiving beams intersect. The received ultrasound contains doppler-shifted components which represent the velocity components of the blood along the direction of the ultrasound beam.

Doppler-shifted components can also be received using a pulsed waveform provided there are sufficient waves at the ultrasonic frequency in each pulse. This allows the principle of range-gating in which the receiving echo amplifier is only turned on for a short time during the receiving phase. This allows reception from one particular depth in the tissue by stepping or sweeping the time of the receiving amplifier gate. Blood flow velocity at a series of points across a blood vessel may be obtained to produce a velocity profile. These pulsed doppler flowmeters may be combined with ultrasonic B-scanners to provide a two-dimensional image of a blood vessel showing only the moving parts of the image (the blood).

The most practical form of ultrasonic blood flowmeter is the continuous wave doppler system with the doppler-shifted components being fed to a zero-crossing detector. This can produce a signal which corresponds approximately to the average blood velocity in the vessel. A slightly more complex version of this allows the independent identification of forward and reverse flow. Forward and reverse flow is represented by the doppler-shifted components above and below the ultrasonic frequency and these can be separated by established methods. The two signals may be fed to separate pen traces or combined in a bi-directional display.

Such devices are mainly used by vascular surgeons. See also Zero-crossing detector, Blood flow meter, Doppler blood flow meter.

Ultrasonic blood pressure monitor $n=3$ $c=4$ $r=1$

Arterial blood pressure has a peak (systolic) pressure occurring when the heart pumps, and a trough (diastolic) just before the next pumping stroke. These two pressures are important indicators of the state of the patient in a number of situations and they are commonly measured by doctors using a mercury-type manometer, an inflatable cuff round the upper arm, and an inflation and deflation device. The cuff pressure corresponds to the systolic pressure when the artery in the arm (brachial artery) just fails to open, and this condition can be detected using a stethoscope on the arm downstream from the cuff. The diastolic pressure is identified as that point when the artery just fails to close. The characteristic sounds (Korotkoff sounds) for these two conditions are recognized by the experienced ear. However, accurate identification is difficult in case of weak pulse, high background noise, or patient movement.

An ultrasonic blood pressure monitor uses the same inflation and deflation sequence to scan the two pressures but the opening of the artery is detected using an ultrasonic doppler device which responds to the movement of the artery wall. A thin ultrasonic transducer is placed on the skin under the inflatable cuff, and coupled to the skin with a jelly to avoid an air gap.

Such devices may be found in operating theatres, wards and some clinics. They may have an automated inflation–deflation sequence to permit repeated measurement and/or recording during anaesthesia or intensive care. The main advantage claimed over acoustic techniques is the high noise immunity and movement noise rejection.

Components of the device are an ultrasonic transducer, an oscillator (e.g. 2 MHz), a high-frequency amplifier, doppler detector and a pattern recognition circuit. Sometimes the pressures are recorded on a paper chart. An example of an ultrasonic blood pressure monitor is the Arteriosonde.

Ultrasonic cleaning bath n=3 c=3

The washing action of detergent or a solvent can be enhanced by the application of ultrasonic waves. Instruments or small components can be cleaned very thoroughly by immersing them in a steel bath (e.g. 25 cm by 15 cm surface area) attached to a high power ultrasonic transducer operating at (say) 50 kHz. This causes rapid shaking of the objects in the bath. The apparatus consists of the bath itself, the transducer (which may be magnetostrictive or piezoelectric) and a high-power oscillator to drive the transducer. These are useful for removing oil or grease, or cleaning blood from intricate instruments.

Ultrasonic diathermy apparatus n=5 c=3,4 r=4,10

Internal heating of tissues can be achieved by the application of a strong ultrasound beam to the skin surface. Ultrasound beams in the low MHz frequencies are commonly used in the physiotherapy department for the treatment of inflammation of joints. The ultrasonic transducer produces a beam of about 1 W/cm^2 which may be applied directly to the skin through a coupling oil or jelly, or the patient (or affected part) may be immersed in water.

It is likely that the beneficial effect of this treatment is due solely to the heat liberated in the tissue as the ultrasonic beam is absorbed, but other mechanisms have been suggested. Most heat is believed to be delivered to the periosteum and hence it is used extensively for treatment of inflamed joint capsules. Most devices deliver a continuous wave, but some have pulsed or pulsating waveforms which may be intended to create a kind of 'ultrasonic massage'.

The apparatus consists of an oscillator, and an amplifier delivering between 1 and 5 W to a resonant piezoelectric transducer. A different transducer is required for each frequency, typically 1, 2 and 3 MHz. At 1 MHz approximately half the energy is released in the first 5 cm. Controls may include intensity and waveform selection.

Ultrasonic massager n=4 c=4 r=4

This is a term sometimes used to describe an ultrasonic treatment unit (ultrasonic diathermy apparatus) used in the physiotherapy department for relieving pain and inflammation. The main effect appears to be heating due to absorption of the waves in the tissue, but there is also the possibility that some of the effect may be due to a sort of 'molecular massage'. An equipment described as an ultrasonic massager may have a variety of treatment regimes involving continuous wave output, pulsed, and pulsating waveforms. See also Ultrasonic diathermy.

Ultrasonic nebulizer n=10 c=3 r=2

Humidification and medication of air or anaesthetic gases may be achieved by using high-intensity ultrasound to break up water, or sterilizing agents, into tiny droplets. There are two main types, those in which the ultrasonic transducer is immersed in fluid from which the mist is projected, and those in which the liquid falls on to the transducer one drop at a time.

Such devices are found in the wards and in the intensive care department. The unit may also incorporate a fan to assist the flow of gases which are being humidified. The humidified gases may be released close to the patient, or ducted directly into the breathing circuit. See also Humidifier.

Ultrasonic scanner n=5 c=6 r=1

Ultrasonic scanners produce echo pictures from within the body. They may be divided into A-scanners, B-scanners (including real-time), M-mode, and doppler instruments. First introduced in the early 1960s they have found widespread use in obstetrics, and for producing images of the liver, kidney, heart, arteries, etc. Development of these devices continues rapidly.

1. A-scanner. A hand-held transducer, applied to the skin, produces a single line on a CRT screen showing the depth of reflecting surfaces. It is used for showing the position of the central structures in the head. It is also used in conjunction with some B-scanners for measurement and setting up.

255

2. B-Scanner. This produces a two-dimensional section scan on a CRT screen which represents a plane of tissue in line with the transducer. The transducer is made to perform a scanning action, to build up the picture from returning echoes. The scanning action may be linear, sector, or compound, and may be produced by hand movement of the transducer, or by motorized rotation or rocking, or produced electronically by switching or phasing pulses to the transducer. Most B-scanners produce moving pictures.

3. M-Mode scanner. A line of dots, representing reflecting surfaces under the transducer, is swept slowly across a long-persistence CRT display so that moving structures can be identified. Such scanners have been used extensively in cardiology for the study of heart valve defects.

4. Doppler Scanner. Information about the movement of blood derived from ultrasonic doppler signals can be assembled into a picture showing only moving parts of the tissue being scanned. Such devices can provide information about vascular disease.

There are other ways in which ultrasonic scanners can be classified, and there are combinations of the above types. Examples are Duplex scanners, which are combinations of B-mode and doppler scanners, C-scanners, transmission scanners, and plan position scanners.

Ultrasonic stethoscope n=5 c=2

This is an incorrect term used in some sales literature for an ultrasonic doppler blood flow detector employed to detect the beating of the foetal heart. See also Doppler foetal heart detector.

Ultrasonic transducer n=1

Ultrasonic waves can be created by the magnetostrictive effect by which the shape of a metal rod is modified by passing an alternating electric current through a coil wound around it. If high frequencies are required, a piezoelectric transducer is more effective.

Some natural materials (e.g. quartz) and some synthetic materials exhibit the piezoelectric effect, by which electric charges appear on their surfaces when they are deformed. Some materials also exhibit the reverse effect by which electric charges applied across the element (crystal) cause it to deform. Thus it can act as a microphone or as a sound generator.

In medical apparatus the transducer element is usually a thin disc or plate of lead zirconate titanate (PZT) of which each face is silvered to form an electrode. It can be made to vibrate at the frequency of an oscillator (as in doppler instruments and physiotherapy apparatus) or if excited by a short electric pulse (as in A- and B-scanners) it will ring at its resonant frequency. The duration of the ringing must be limited to provide a short pulse of sound, and this is achieved by attaching sound-absorbing material to the back of the element. The front face is applied to the skin through focusing and impedance matching layers and a coupling oil or jelly.

Doppler instruments commonly make use of separate crystals for transmit and receive, which are angled together so that reception of echoes is most effective at a chosen depth. Pulse-echo equipment usually employs the same crystal for both functions with some form of focusing lens.

Multi-element transducers are now common in real-time B-scanners. The piezoelectric element is divided into many parallel strips. In real-time linear array scanners there may be 64 parallel elements stretching 10 cm or so, and these are used in groups so that the active area of the crystal is electronically moved along, simulating movement of a square transducer. In electronically steered array scanners each element is driven at a different time so that the ultrasound beam may be made to point in (or receive from) any direction. Focusing of the transmitted wave, and dynamic focusing during the receiving phase can be achieved in a similar way.

Ultrasonic treatment unit n=4 c=4 r=4,10

Heat can be generated within the body by the absorption of ultrasound delivered through the skin from a piezoelectric transducer. The frequency employed is usually between 1 and 3 MHz and the intensity about 1 W/cm^2 at the skin. Such devices are used for the treatment of injury, pain, inflammation, etc. in the physiotherapy department. See Ultrasonic diathermy for further details.

Ultraviolet recorder n=3 c=4,5

Signals which change rapidly (e.g. above 50 Hz maximum frequency) may not be accurately recorded using a pen recorder. This problem can be overcome by using a low-inertia galvanometer system. In the ultraviolet recorder ultraviolet light is directed through a slit and lens system on to a tiny mirror mounted within a small galvanometer coil in a narrow tube placed in a strong magnetic field. As the current in the coil varies in time with the signal to be measured the mirror swings so directing the beam of ultraviolet light on to a moving paper strip. A number of different signals may be recorded simultaneously but this may cause problems of identification of each channel if they cross over.

Ultraviolet recorders may be used wherever high-speed operation is required. They are sometimes used to record electromyograms (EMG).

Ultraviolet treatment lamp n=5 c=3 r=4

This produces electromagnetic radiation of wavelengths between 180 and 400 nm. For descriptive purposes the ultraviolet spectrum is divided into the following ranges:

UVA	315–400 nm
UVB	280–315 nm
UVC	below 280 nm

The lamps are usually high-pressure mercury-quartz arc in a housing with a quartz window, cooled by either water flow or air blast. Fluorescent tubes are also available which produce light in the ultraviolet region.

They are mainly used in the treatment of diseases of the skin, tuberculosis, ulcerations, rheumatic conditions, and some childhood diseases. Vitamin D is produced in the skin in the presence of ultraviolet light and this effect has been used in the treatment of rickets in children. Ultraviolet light is toxic and needs to be monitored, particularly since the efficiency of the lamps decreases with time. The standard dose is the minimal erythemic dose or MED. This is the dose at which the skin shows a mild reddening 24 hours after the treatment.

A special type of mercury-vapour lamp used in the physiotherapy department is the Kromayer lamp which has a water-cooling system, and the rays actually pass through the water, so as to remove infrared radiation. The advantage of this type of lamp is that it can be applied directly to the area to be treated rather than operating remotely.

Urethroscope n=5 c=3 r=4

This is a small rigid telescope which may be passed up the urethra to view the state of the urethral wall and prostate gland. It differs from a cystoscope because it has an end rather than a side view. This type of endoscope, sometimes called a panendoscope, does not normally have extra channels for the passage of surgical instruments, although it must be possible to infuse fluids to create a small viewing space at the end. See also Endoscope.

Urilos electronic nappy n=3 c=3

Investigation of the quantity or pattern of urine loss in cases of urinary incontinence may be conducted using an electronic recording system. The transducer for this is a disposable 'nappy' (diaper) impregnated with common salt and including sewn-in aluminium strip electrodes. The change in electrical impedance is recorded in response to urine leakage into the nappy.

Urinometer r=6

A device for measuring and electrically recording the volume and rate of urine output from a patient in intensive care, via a urethral catheter. One such device senses the pressure head developed at the bottom of a narrow vessel. The vessel empties periodically and a computer record is made of the volumes emptied. In general, manual recording of urine output is considered satisfactory.

Urodynamic apparatus n=1 c=6

Some disorders of the bladder and urethra, especially those resulting in urinary incontinence or retention, are investigated in a special urodynamic clinic which may be in the urology, gynaecology or X-ray department. The main apparatus is a multichannel chart recorder with additional equipment which may include a uroflowmeter, profilometer, catheter puller, and X-ray fluoroscope. The multichannel recorder may include the functions of a cystometer, urethral pressure profile recorder and electromyograph.

Typical urodynamic tests may include:

1. Cystometry. The bladder is filled through a urethral catheter while recording the pressure generated within the bladder. Often the net contribution to pressure from the bladder muscle itself is recorded by electronically subtracting the pressure in the rectum from the total pressure in the bladder.
2. Urometry. The flow rate during normal bladder emptying is plotted on the chart recorder. The total volume voided is also calculated.
3. Profilometry. A plot of pressure along the urethra is recorded using an external pressure transducer with a slow infusion through the urethral catheter, or a tiny pressure transducer may be mounted on the recording catheter. The catheter may be moved along the urethra using a catheter puller.
4. Urethral pressure transmission tests. Pressures recorded from the rectum are subtracted from the pressures detected at various points along the urethra during coughing or straining. The relative changes in the two pressures are used to assess the ability of the urethra to close in response to high abdominal pressures.
5. Fluid bridge test. Penetration of urine into the upper part of the urethra during coughing and straining can be detected by pressure measurements, or by leakage into a catheter opening into the urethra, or by electrical impedance measurements between two metal rings mounted on the urethral catheter.
6. Electromyography. The action of muscles in and around the urethra may

be recorded during the tests using electrodes mounted on the urethral catheter, using a needle electrode inserted into the muscles, or from surface electrodes on the perineum.

7. Cystoscopy. Direct viewing of the inside of the bladder and urethra via a cystoscope or urethroscope can sometimes provide additional information about urodynamic function.

8. Fluoroscopy. The bladder is filled with an X-ray contrast medium and viewed during filling, during straining and coughing, and during emptying. Diagnostic information is obtained from the shape of the bladder base and from visualization of the entry of contrast medium into the urethra.

In many cases a video tape recording is made of the X-ray image of the bladder and urethra overlayed with the pressure, EMG and flow recordings.

Uroflowmeter n=1 c=4

A recording of urine flow during bladder emptying is sometimes performed to investigate disorders of bladder control. The subject urinates into the uroflowmeter and a recording of flow rate and volume voided is made. The device may work by:

1. Recording the height of a column of urine in a tall measuring cylinder. The height of the column is detected by measuring pressure at the bottom, or by recording electrical conductance or capacitance using a pair of long electrodes immersed in the urine. In both cases the flow rate is calculated by electronic differentiation.

2. The urine is directed on to a rotating disc with vanes. The drag on the motor rotating the disc is detected electronically and the flow rate is calculated from this.

3. The urine is directed on to a pressure plate which detects the force of the flow and the flow rate is calculated from this force.

4. The flow is directed into a series of cuvettes. The volume in each cuvette is calculated and the flow profile is plotted.

Such devices are used in the urodynamic clinic which may be situated in the urology, gynaecology or X-ray department.

V

Vacuum control valve r=2

This is a bleed valve sometimes fitted between the source of vacuum (pump, pipeline, injector or venturi) and the suction jar which admits air to reduce the degree of vacuum. They are used in medical suction units and machines.

Vacuum pump r=2

Many types of vacuum, or suction, pumps exist in hospitals. They are found in medical suction machines, but also in some analytical apparatus, and they may be piston types, diaphragm pumps, rotating vane types, or bellows. They may be motor driven, pneumatically operated or foot operated.

Vacuum unit n=300 c=1,3 r=2

Although this term may be applied to any vacuum pump, it is more commonly an alternative name for a (medical) suction unit or machine, usually attached to a vacuum pipeline.

Vaporizer n=50 c=2 r=2

Although one might expect this term to be applied to any form of vaporizer, perhaps including humidifiers and nebulizers, it is normally reserved for devices for producing vapour from volatile anaesthetic agents such as ether, chloroform, halothane, etc. These are used to introduce such agents into the inspired gases during anaesthesia. Gases are blown through, over the surface, or over a wick of the volatile liquids to produce vapour.

Earlier types were simple bubble-through devices but modern vaporizers are complex with relatively accurate calibration and temperature compensation, usually with the aid of a thermostatically controlled valve.

They usually fit on to the back bar of the anaesthetic machine so that the gas mixtures from the flowmeters can pass through, collecting the vapour. Although there are some types which can take a variety of anaesthetic agents, the trend is to provide temperature compensated and calibrated units for single agents. They consist of terminal connections on to the back bar, a reservoir, wick or other dispersing mechanism, a temperature-compensating mechanism and a control system.

Types which may be found include the copper kettle, draw over, Fluotec, Abingdon, Oxford, Enfluratec, Pentec, and others. Special 'draw over' types which provide a very low resistance to the flow of gas are made for intermittent (demand) flow apparatus, for dental anaesthesia, and for circle rebreathing circuits.

Vascular dilator n=1 c=3,4

To facilitate venous puncture with difficult-to-locate vessels it is normal to apply a pressure cuff to the upper arm, and to ask the patient to clench his fist. The vessels can be further dilated by the application of surface heat. Machines exist to provide all three of these stimuli simultaneously with a special hand-grip, a pressure cuff for the upper arm and a heating pad over the lower arm.

Vectorcardiograph n=1 c=5 r=9

Electrical signals from the heart are normally presented as a graph of voltage against time. The voltages developed along the various axes of the heart are recorded using a set of lead configurations which are selected in turn. However, more information can be derived from a vectorcardiogram (VCG) which can deliver a three-dimensional picture of the orientation and magnitude of the cardiac electrical vector throughout the cardiac cycle. In practice a two-dimensional image is displayed for each of the orthogonal planes.

A system of electrode positions has been developed to collect the X, Y and Z components of the ECG and any two of these can be fed through amplifiers to the X and Y deflection plates of a cathode ray tube. The ECG cycle is therefore presented as a loop on the screen representing the path of the electrical vector. The three possible planes of the vectorcardiogram may be shown in sequence and be photographed or collected in a computer memory for slow rate output to an X–Y recorder. Normal and abnormal patterns of the VCG loop are well documented.

Venous occlusion plethysmograph n=1 c=3 r=6

An inflatable cuff placed around the upper part of a limb, inflated so as to prevent the return of venous blood to the heart (e.g. to 50 mmHg) but not to obstruct arterial blood, causes swelling of the limb due to the inflow of blood. The rate of inflow of blood to the limb (limb perfusion rate) can therefore be detected from the rate of increase in limb volume over the first few heartbeats.

As the venous return is occluded, the limb volume may be sensed in a variety of ways including strain gauge plethysmography and electrical impedance plethysmography. Plethysmography means recording volume changes.

Such a device might be used in the study of vascular disease.

Venous pressure monitor r=9

Measurements of venous pressure are an important aid to the physician for determining the function of the capillary bed and the right heart. The venous pressure has little pulse and so a steady state measurement is normally adequate. This is achieved by making a puncture into a vein using a large bore needle, and passing a plastic tube through it which is advanced to the correct position before the needle is removed. The tube is connected to a short saline-filled tube which is held vertical against a calibrated backing strip, or it may be connected to a high-sensitivity pressure transducer.

The most common venous pressure measurement is the central venous pressure, which is measured in one of the large veins returning to the heart, or in the right atrium. The reference level of the pressure is the right atrium, and the measurement is used widely in intensive care to monitor therapy of heart dysfunction, shock, hypo- or hyper-volaemic states, or circulatory failure. It is used as a guide to determine the amount of liquid the patient should receive.

Ventilator n=50 c=1,4 r=2,6

In medical work this term usually refers to a breathing machine for providing assisted or artificial ventilation of the lungs. It can thus mean a resuscitator for emergency use, a body respirator (e.g. cuirass), or lung ventilator (see Intermittent positive pressure ventilator). In any form its function is to assist or take over from the spontaneous respiratory effort of the patient. These are used during anaesthesia (where muscle relaxants impair natural breathing), in intensive care for life support, and during emergency resuscitation.

Ventilator alarm n=20 c=3 r=2,6

To detect failure of a lung ventilator or accidental disconnection in the patient circuit, it is wise to employ an alarm device to show if the pressure in the breathing circuit goes outside preset limits, or if the machine fails to provide the correct ventilation cycle. This type of device is useful during anaesthesia, and in intensive care, where the ventilator must operate for long periods without close supervision.

Vibromassager n=2 c=2

Many types of vibromassage apparatus exist. The most common type is used in the physiotherapy department to automate the application of massage. It is usually hand held and delivers a rapid shaking motion through a soft applicator. The device is usually electrically operated and contains a motor with an eccentric weight, but may include a different type of shaker. Effective treatment is claimed for arthritis, lumbago, sciatica, varicose veins, varicose ulcers, impaired circulation, and dispersal of adipose tissue.

Visual display unit n=20

Modern computers are usually accessed through a visual display unit (VDU) which contains a television-type cathode ray tube and drive electronics, a key board and often enough internal memory to store a full screen of information. They are sometimes called computer terminals although this implies additional abilities such as screen editing, limited storage of information and encoding of information for transmission and reception. They are found in many situations throughout the hospital from patient records departments where they may be linked to a central management computer, or to pathology laboratories where they may be linked to a scientific computer.

Visual field analyser

The subject places his chin on a rest, and the eye to be tested is focused on a white disc in the centre of the apparatus. A second fixation target is slowly moved in from the periphery of vision and the subject indicates when he first sees it. By moving the second target in from different directions it is possible to plot isopters on a graph of visual field. Refinements include automatic mapping and circuits to detect if the eye wanders from the main fixation target. The device is also known as a perimeter.

Vital signs monitor n=5 c=4

Recent improvements in signal processing techniques have enabled the development of non-invasive blood pressure metering of adequate reliability for anaesthetized and tranquil patients. Blood pressure metering is achieved by a normal cuff method, usually sensing the arterial pulsations via the cuff inflating tube.

It has become common to include a non-invasive blood pressure monitor which can display mean blood pressure, average systolic and average diastolic pressure, pulse rate, patient temperature and sometimes breathing rate in a single instrument, and this is called a vital signs monitor by some manufacturers.

Vitalograph n=3 c=3 r=2

This is a trade name which is sometimes applied to all bellows types of spirometer. It consists of a large hinged-type bellows in a box. The lower side of the bellows is fixed, while the upper part operates a pen which moves over a chart to indicate the volume of gas inside. The subject blows into the bellows after a deep breath and a graph is produced of volume exhaled against time. From the resulting graph the forced vital capacity (FVC) can be read as well as the forced expiratory volume (FEV). The peak flow rate can also be deduced.

Such devices are found in a lung function laboratory for assessing the performance of the lungs.

Vocoder r=4

Vocoders attempt to provide speech information via tactile or visual routes. Speech is analysed into frequency components and the relative amplitudes of these operate tactile or visual displays. Tactile vocoders usually employ a bank of filters and present the amplitude of each frequency band via vibrators placed on the skin. Tactile actuators suffer from problems of interaction and masking by other tactile inputs.

Visual vocoders may be coupled to a series of lights related to each frequency range or to a CRT display. Success with these devices has unfortunately been poor, but the potential exists for improved processing and display using computers.

Voiscope n=1 c=4

This is an instrument based on the laryngograph employing surface-mounted electrodes adjacent to the glottis and providing an electrical analogue of the movement of the larynx. The voiscope provides a visual display of the speech fundamental frequency information on an oscilloscope screen and this can be used to assist the patient to correct and reinforce voice, rhythm and intonation patterns. Gross larynx movement may also be detected to observe and record the slow laryngeal adjustments which precede and accompany phonation. The device may be used in the speech therapy department under supervision, or by the patient alone using programmed material.

VOLUMETRIC INFUSION PUMP

Volumetric infusion pump n=40 c=3,4

Very accurate flow rates of intravenous fluids may be delivered by passing the fluid through a bi-directional motor-driven syringe (a cassette unit). The cassette is a disposable element which fits on to a drive shaft or other mechanism and connects into the giving set tube. Fluid is drawn into one side of the cassette while the other side of the plunger is discharging through the intravenous cannula. These are used throughout the hospital, particularly in intensive care areas. The advantage of these types of devices over peristaltic pumps, or over infusion controllers, is that there can be no error due to incorrect placement or malfunction of the drop counting detector. They do however require alarm circuitry to detect excessive back pressure, or the presence of air in the giving set when the reservoir bag is exhausted.

Walking platform n=1 c=5

Walking patterns may be assessed for diagnostic purposes, but more commonly for studying the functioning of artificial hips and knees, artificial legs, and external support mechanisms (orthoses). The apparatus used is likely to include a walking platform, also known as a force plate, which consists of a metal plate held by a strong suspension in a frame with strain gauges, to measure the forces applied by the foot in three orthogonal directions as well as the rotational forces.

The apparatus may come with the necessary strain gauge amplifiers, and with a computer and programs to resolve the forces and moments, and to provide graphical display of the results. Such a device might be used in the orthopaedic surgery or limb fitting department.

Wall suction unit n=300 c=1 r=2

These are medical suction units intended to plug into the wall suction supply (piped suction). They include a connector to mate with the wall suction outlet, a gauge to show the vacuum, a control valve, filters and a reservoir.

Warble-tone audiometer n=1 c=3

Audiology and hearing aid departments often use free-field tests (as opposed to using headphones) for diagnostic and hearing aid fitting purposes. Free-field tests should ideally be conducted in an acoustic booth or audiometric room having a low reverberation time and walls with a high sound-absorbing quality, so that the space appears to be a free field. In all but the highest quality audiometric room, there is a problem with standing waves when using single-frequency test tones. This occurs when the distance between any two surfaces in the room is a multiple of the wavelength of the test tone and results in areas of high and low-intensity sound, reducing the potential accuracy of the method. One way of reducing this problem is to use a warble-tone audiometer which produces test tones with rapidly fluctuating frequency (warble tones) instead of pure tones. A warble-tone generator is often an accessory for a pure-tone audiometer.

Water bath n=50 c=2

This is usually a small steel bath filled with water which is heated by an electric element controlled by a temperature sensor in the water and usually having a motor-driven stirrer to ensure even temperature distribution throughout the water. These are used to provide controlled temperature for chemical reactions in test tubes or flasks partially immersed in the water, or for heating blood or other fluids (e.g. peritoneal dialysis fluids) which are to be passed into the body. They are also used as caloric tanks for feeding water of a known temperature into the ear during vestibulometric tests. Because of the presence of water, the electrical requirements of such devices are more stringent than normal and an overtemperature cut-out is also required in case of failure of the primary control mechanism.

Water bed/mattress n=10 c=3

In cases where it is very important that the patient is supported without applying large pressures to the skin (e.g. in burns cases) the bed may consist of a large tank of warmed water covered by a plastic sheet. The patient floats as if in water but is kept dry. An alternative version is a thin mattress consisting of a double sheet of plastic welded together to provide two separate channels for the water to pass through. A ripple effect is achieved by directing the warm water through one channel for a few minutes, and then through the other so that the patient is supported on different parts of the mattress in the two phases of the cycle thus avoiding prolonged pressure on any point on the body.

Typical parameters for a ripple heat mattress and controller might be heating from 20 to 37°C in 15 minutes from a 2 litre reservoir tank, and delivering a flow rate of 45 l/h in the ripple mode and twice this in the non-ripple mode. The ripple cycle might be 6 minutes.

Water manometer n=20 r=2

A vertical glass tube, or a U-tube makes an excellent manometer suitable for the calibration of pressure measuring apparatus, or to measure slowly changing pressures such as the central venous pressure or bladder pressure. The theory of operation is identical to the mercury manometer but there is a scale factor difference of 13.6 since water is a lighter fluid. Greater sensitivity can be achieved by inclining the tube. In this way the distance the surface of the water must move to register a particular vertical rise is greater.

Water manometers are normally calibrated in cm H_2O which is convenient when using water filled tubing, since errors of level normally cancel out. Water manometers would normally be found in intensive care applications (for CVP pressure) and as calibration units wherever pressures are measured using electric manometers (theatres, high dependency wards, urodynamic clinics, cardiac catheter laboratories).

Water softener

Water softeners are resin bed ion exchangers. They contain a cation resin bed which exchanges the cation sodium for the cations calcium and magnesium in the water, both of which are harmful to patients on haemodialysis. The resin bed exhausts when all the sodium ions have been exchanged. The resin bed can be regenerated by back-flushing with a brine solution. A water softener is also used as a pre-treatment for a reverse osmosis unit. Water softeners are used with haemodialysis machines in hard water areas.

Waters canister n=5 c=1 r=2

This is a carbon dioxide absorber containing soda-lime used in rebreathing anaesthetic circuits. It connects between the breathing bag and the facepiece or endotracheal tube. One advantage of this in-line type of absorber is that it can be sterilized relatively easily after use on infected patients. Defects of such 'to and fro' absorbers are water logging due to condensation, channelling of the gases (thus defeating the absorber) due to shake down of the granules, and imperfect containment of the soda-lime leading to inhalation of some of the dust.

Wax bath n=2 c=2 r=10

This is usually a thermostatically controlled heating vessel typically 25 cm by 50 cm in which a wax is heated to approximately 40–44°C. Heating may be direct or via a water jacket. Hot wax treatment is one of a number of methods used in the physiotherapy department for applying heat to the body. The heated wax is transferred to a secondary vessel (bowl) and is then transferred to the area being treated. In some cases the patient immerses the limb being treated into the bowl and lifts it out so that some wax solidifies on the skin. The process is repeated several times until a thick coating of wax is formed. The wax is a poor conductor of heat and releases the heat slowly into the limb as it solidifies.

Wax baths are also used in the preparation of ear moulds and further details may be found under that heading.

Weighing bed n=2 c=4

In dialysis, intensive care, and in the treatment of patients suffering from burns, a bed weighing system is useful for monitoring weight changes. Patients suffering from fluid loss or undergoing fluid correction can be managed better by monitoring the patient's weight while the patient is in bed.

The instrument consists of four load cells mounted in the legs of the bed, or placed under the wheels, and a central control unit which calculates and displays the total weight of the bed. Changes in total weight can then be monitored.

Well counter r=3

This is a special type of scintillation counter in which the scintillation crystal is shaped in the form of a well to receive a small vial containing the sample whose radioactivity is to be counted. The crystal must be covered in a thin aluminium can to exclude light, and so they are only suitable for counting relatively high radiation energy (greater than 20 keV of gamma rays). They are used in an autogamma counter in conjunction with an automatic sample changer.

Whirlpool bath r=4

One of the many possible devices for applying heat treatment for pain, spasm or inflammation is the whirlpool bath. Generalized heating of the patient or a limb is provided by the water and the whirlpool action reduces the weight supported by the limb undergoing treatment. Such devices would not commonly be found in hospitals but more in special treatment centres.

Williams filter r=2

A bacterial filter for use in anaesthetic and lung ventilator airways.

Wisconsin test cassette n=1 c=3,4

This is a special X-ray film cassette which produces a pattern on the X-ray film caused by differing attenuations through various thicknesses of copper in the cassette. The pattern produced allows calculation of the kilovoltage of the X-ray set.

A general term for this device is a penetrameter, and more details are given under that heading.

Wright peak flowmeter n=5 c=2 r=2,6

A hand-held device into which the patient blows with maximum force after a deep breath and which shows the peak flow rate reached during the forced expiration. The device operates by the air deflecting a vane against a spiral spring. As the vane moves further round the dial, more escape holes are uncovered. There is a ratchet to hold the vane in the furthest position reached, and a release/reset button is provided. Typical peak expiratory flow rate (PEFR) for an adult male is 7 l/min. Other (electronic) types of peak flowmeter exist. It is used in the lung function laboratory.

Wright's respiration monitor/meter n=10 c=3 r=2,6

An electronic integrator of gas flow through a transducer which fits into the anaesthetic or ventilator breathing circuit. The scale can be set to indicate either tidal volume or minute volume. Tidal volume range is 200–1500 ml and minute volume is from 4 to 30 l/min. The transducer is similar to that in the Wright's respirometer but it detects the rotation of the vane by an optical method. This would be used by anaesthetists during anaesthesia or intensive care when using a lung ventilator.

Wright's respirometer n=30 c=2 r=2,6

A gas volume meter for use in the breathing circuit of an anaesthetic machine or ventilator which works by directing the breathing gases through oblique slots in a small cylinder enclosing a small vane which is made to rotate. The spindle on which the vane is mounted drives a gear train connected to a pointer which moves over a dial indicating the volume of gas passed. Gases which flow back through the device do not register since they enter along the axis of the vane spindle. A key feature of the Wright's respirometer is a mercurial seal between the measuring chamber and the gear train which prevents moisture penetrating the mechanism. It has controls to lock the mechanism and to reset the pointer to zero. The dial has an additional scale driven by a further gear so that accumulated gas flow is indicated. Some errors occur at high and low flows but these tend to cancel out under respiratory flow patterns. The Drager volumeter is somewhat similar.

X

Xenograft r=4

This is an implant transferred from an animal of different species (sometimes called a heterograft). This is most commonly encountered as the tissue heart valve. A substitute heart valve (porcine bioprosthesis) may be made from the natural valve of a specially bred pig. The valve is removed from the pig and carefully sewn on to a metal or plastic ring which is covered with a woven fabric (often Dacron), which can then be sewn in place of a diseased heart valve. These valves provide good flow characteristics compared with mechanical (ball or disc) valves but introduce different problems of tissue preparation and antigenic reaction.

Xeroradiography apparatus n=1 c=6

Instant radiographs can be produced by the same process as used in the Xerox photocopier. A thin semiconductive layer of amorphous selenium is charged up to a high voltage (600–1200 V). When this layer is exposed to light (or X-rays) the exposed areas become conductive and transfer the charge to an aluminium plate beneath. An aerosol of negatively charged particles is then attracted on to the remaining charged areas, and these particles are then baked on to paper. This paper then has the X-ray image without further development.

Although there is an advantage in having instant radiographs the technique has not become popular because the radiation exposure required is much higher than with conventional radiographs, and there are a number of defects in the image which are well known in photocopiers, such as excessive contrast and edge enhancement. The high contrast can, however, be useful for imaging areas of low subject contrast, such as breasts, soft tissues, calcifications, and hair-line fractures.

X-ray film cassette r=7

Although X-rays will produce an image on photographic film, the effect is inefficient, and most of the rays pass straight through. In practice, X-ray film is exposed by light emitted by fluorescent (intensifying) screens held in contact with the front and back of the film in a special cassette.

The light-tight film cassette is made up of several layers. There is a thin plastic sheet on the side which faces the patient and X-ray tube, and beneath this there is a thin fluorescent layer. This layer absorbs the X-rays more strongly than the film and produces a fluorescent image which is transposed to the photographic emulsion on the upper side of the film. X-ray film is dual sided, and so a second fluorescent layer (thicker than the first) is beneath the film. There may be a lead foil layer next, which is particularly important if cassettes are stacked in the magazine of a rapid cassette changer.

It is most important that there is intimate contact between the film and the fluorescent screens if a sharp image is to formed. Some cassettes include a secondary radiation grid for situations where a moving grid is not being used.

X-ray set $n = 12$ $c = 5,6,7,8$ $r = 7$

Therapeutic X-ray sets exist for the treatment of skin and superficial disorders, and these consist of an X-ray generator and suitable positioning and beam collimating equipment. However, the majority of X-ray apparatus is for the production of images on film or video screens for diagnostic purposes.

All diagnostic sets consist of an X-ray source (tube) and a detection system which may be photographic film, an image intensifier, or photomultiplier tube, usually with X-ray to optical ray conversion by a fluorescent screen or scintillator. Sets may be designed to undertake a single type of examination, such as dental imaging, or may be generalized sets able to perform single film X-rays, cine, video, tomography, bi-plane etc. Some of these variations are listed below:

1. General purpose. Able to take single films. The unit usually has a couch with the tube mounted above, and the film below. The tube can usually be moved to various positions and angles including the horizontal position for chest films, in which case the cassette and Bucky are in a separate stand.
2. Fluoroscopes. Moving picture images can be obtained using an image intensifier and cine, or video system. Many sets can perform fluoroscopy as well as single films.
3. Cardioangiography sets. Fluoroscopic images and films can be produced, often in two planes simultaneously.
4. Tomographic units. Films showing a single plane within the body can be produced by rotating or moving the tube and film simultaneously so that only images from the chosen plane remain in focus throughout the movement.
5. Dental sets. Small pieces of X-ray film are placed inside the mouth and low-power X-rays applied through the cheeks. Sometimes the X-ray

273

source is placed inside the mouth and the film wrapped around the jaw (Panoral X-ray).

6. Panoral sets. A view through all of the teeth can be obtained by placing a low-power X-ray source inside the mouth and detecting the results on a film wrapped around the jaw.

7. Mammography sets. Good contrast in the soft tissues of the breast can be obtained using a special X-ray tube with a molybdenum anode which produces a narrow band of soft X-rays.

8. CT Scanners. A narrow beam of X-rays is scanned across a section of the body and the X-ray absorption of each point within the scanning plane is determined and displayed by computer.

X-ray therapy apparatus n=2 c=6 r=4

High-energy X-rays are used to treat cancer, since some cancer cells are more susceptible to damage from electromagnetic radiation than ordinary cells. The energy of the X-rays (usually expressed in kilovoltage) determines the depth of penetration. Thus for superficial X-rays (suitable for skin treatment) 50–150 kV may be used. Conventional X-ray generators may be used to generate up to 500 kV rays. Higher energies require a linear accelerator or betatron.

X-ray tube r=7

The X-rays are produced by two processes. Electrons may collide with the nuclear field around an atom, losing part of their energy, producing X-ray energies up to the maximum energy of the incident electrons, or electrons are ejected from the target atom which, when replaced, release energy dependent upon the atomic structure of that atom. Thus the energy spectrum produced will contain both continuous and line spectra.

The X-ray tube as used in diagnostic X-ray apparatus consists of an evacuated envelope containing a source of focused electrons (cathode) directed on to an anode which has a very high melting point and a high atomic number. The anode becomes very hot and so for all but the lowest power units this problem is dealt with by rotating the anode at high speed (3000 to 10 000 rev/min) to distribute the heat. The target material on the anode is usually tungsten (melting point 3370°C, atomic number 74) but molybdenum is also used for low power (e.g. mammography) sets.

The assembly, which one sees containing the tube, also contains terminals for the very high voltages applied between anode and cathode (up to 150 kV), and an air or oil-cooling system on high-power sets. There is also the rotating mechanism for the anode and special filters, cones or collimators, and diaphragms, making up the X-ray window.

X-ray tubes have a limited life.

274

X–Y recorder n=3 c=3,4 r=3

This is a paper chart recorder for producing graphs of one variable against another. It has a separate signal amplifier to drive the pen in the X (horizontal) direction and the Y (vertical) direction. Both are normally potentiometric mechanisms to achieve a wide span. Such recorders are used in the audiology department for plotting acoustic impedance change against outer ear pressure, and for other applications to plot one variable against another.

Z

Zero-crossing ratemeter r=1,9

The velocity of blood flowing in a vessel can be calculated from the doppler-shifted reflections of a continuous-wave ultrasound beam, transmitted through it from a point outside the body. A major problem arises because in addition to the pulsatile nature of the blood flow, many different doppler-shifted frequencies are received due to the differing velocities flowing at each point across the vessel (flow at the centre is normally faster than near the walls).

There are two main methods of dealing with this problem. One is to apply a complete frequency analysis to the signals (using a spectrograph), and the second is to derive an approximate figure for average blood velocity using a zero-crossing ratemeter. This counts the rate at which the signal passes through the zero level and the result is a mean velocity which can be recorded on a strip chart, but does not exactly reflect the flow pattern.

Such devices are used in the more basic types of doppler blood flowmeters for estimating the quality of flow through peripheral blood vessels during the assessment of vascular disease, and in more complex types, including pulsed-wave doppler velocity meters, where accuracy is greater in view of the smaller sampling volume.

Appendix 1

List of abbreviations

AIUM	American Institute for Ultrasound in Medicine
ALU	Arithmetic and logic unit (computers)
ASCII	American Standard Code for Information Interchange (computers)
Bq	Becquerel (1 nuclear disintegration/s)
CAPD	Continuous ambulatory peritoneal dialysis
CAT	Computerized axial tomography (X-ray scanners)
CMRR	Common mode rejection ratio (amplifiers)
Ci	Curie (3.7×10^{10} nuclear disintegrations/s)
CPAP	Constant positive airway pressure
CRT	Cathode ray tube
CVP	Central venous pressure
CW	Continuous wave (e.g. of doppler ultrasound)
DHSS	Department of Health and Social Security (UK)
ECG	Electrocardiogram
ECochG	Electrocochleogram
ECT	Electroconvulsive therapy
EEG	Electroencephalogram
EKG	Electrocardiogram (American)
ELCB	Earth leakage circuit breaker
EMG	Electromyogram
ENG	Electronystagmogram/electroneurogram
EOG	Electro-oculogram
ENT	Ear nose and throat (specialization of surgery)
ERA	Electric response audiometry
ERG	Electroretinogram
ERP	Early receptor potential (of eyes)
ERV	Expiratory reserve volume (lungs)
eV	Electron volt (unit of radiation energy)
FEF	Forced expiratory flow (lungs)
FEV1	Forced expiratory volume after 1 second (of lungs)
FGF	Fresh gas flow (anaesthetic machine)
FM	Frequency modulation (radio and tape recorders)
FRC	Functional residual capacity (lungs)
FVC	Forced vital capacity (of lungs)
GM tube	Geiger-Müller tube
HDU	High dependency unit
IEC	International Electrotechnical Commission
I:E ratio	Inspiratory to expiratory ratio (lung ventilator)
IMV	Intermittent mandatory ventilation
IPPV	Intermittent positive pressure ventilation

APPENDIX I

ISG	Indocyanine green (dye dilution)
IV	Intravenous
kV	Kilovoltage (X-ray set)
MeV	Mega electron volts (energy of ionizing radiation)
NEEP	Negative end expiratory pressure
PAM	Post auricular myogenic (response)
PAO_2	Arterial oxygen pressure
PaO_2	Alveolar oxygen pressure
pCO_2	Partial pressure of carbon dioxide
PEEP	Positive end expiratory pressure
PEFR	Peak expiratory flow rate (lung function)
pO_2	Partial pressure of oxygen
PZT	Lead zirconate titanate (ultrasonic transducers)
RAM	Random access memory (computers)
RIA	Radioimmunoassay
ROM	Read only memory (computers)
RV	Residual volume (lung function)
SVR	Slow vertex response (electric response audiometry)
TENS	Transcutaneous electrical neural stimulation
TGC	Time–gain compensation (ultrasonic scanners)
TLD	Thermoluminescent dosimetry (radiation protection)
TM	Time–motion (ultrasonic scanner)
VC	Vital capacity (lung function)
VCG	Vectorcardiogram
VT	Tidal volume (lung function)
VDU	Visual display unit (for computer)
VER	Visual evoked response (of sight)
VEP	Visual evoked potential (of sight)

Appendix 2

This appendix list entries considered relevant to the following subjects:

Anaesthesia
Audiology and speech therapy
Cardiology
Dialysis
Electrical, electronics and computing
Ionizing radiation

Lung function testing
Medical laboratory equipment
Miscellaneous medical equipment
Physiotherapy
Surgery
Ultrasonics

Entries relevant to anaesthesia

Absorber
Air entrainment valve
Air viva respirator/resuscitator
Airway
Aldasorber
Ambu 'E' valve
Ambu facepiece
Ambu respirator/resuscitator
Anaesthetic circuit
Anaesthetic machine
Analgesia apparatus
Anemometer
Aneroid pressure gauges
Apnoea alarm/monitor
Artificial lung
Artificial nose
Artificial thumb
Aspirator
Atomizer
Ayres T-piece
Back bar
Bag squeezer
Ball float meter
Basket anaesthetic machine
Belt respirator
Blow-off valve
Bodok seals
Body respirator
Bosun oxygen failure warning device
Bourdon gauge (manometer)

Boyles bottle (vaporizer)
Boyles machine
Brachial stethoscope
Breathing circuit
Breathing machine
Breathing tube/hose
Bull-nosed cylinder valves
Cabinet ventilator
Capnometer/capnograph
Carbon dioxide absorber
Cardiff swivel
Catheter mount
Central venous pressure (cvp) monitor
Cerebral function monitor
Circle absorber
Closed circuit
Copper kettle (vaporizer)
Cuirass ventilator
Demand flow analgesia apparatus
Drager volumeter
Draw-over apparatus
Draw-over vaporizer
Drinker apparatus
East Radcliffe ventilator
Electroanaesthesia apparatus
Electroanalgesia apparatus
Elephant tubing
Emerson cuirass ventilator
Endobronchial tube
Endotracheal connector

Endotracheal tube
Entonox apparatus
Expiratory valve
Face mask
Facepiece
Feed mount
Fleisch tube
Flowmeter
Fluotec
Fraser Sweatman pin safety system
Fuel cell oxygen analyser
Gas cylinder
Gas mixing valve
Goldman inhaler
Goldman vaporizer
Haldane apparatus
Head harness
Heidbrink valve
Humidifier
Infrared carbon dioxide analyser
Injector suction unit
Intermittent blower ventilator
Intermittent flow apparatus
Intermittent positive pressure ventilator (IPPV)
Iron lung
Isolette negative pressure apparatus
Jackson Rees paediatric T-tube
Laryngoscope
Liquid oxygen supply
Low-resistance vaporizer
Lung ventilator
Magill attachment
Manley ventilator
Mapleson breathing circuit
Marshall's indicator
Mass spectroscope/spectrograph
McKesson breathing circuits
McKesson expiratory valve
McKesson inhaler
Mechanical thumb ventilator
Medical compressed air
Minute volume divider
Nebulizer
Oesophageal stethoscope
Open circuit
Open drop mask
Oscillometer
Oscillotonometer
Oxygen analyser

Oxygen bypass (flush) control
Oxygen failure warning device
Paramagnetic oxygen analyser
Patient circuit
PEEP valve
Peripheral nerve stimulator
Pin-index system
Pinkerton cuirass ventilator
Piped medical gas supply
Pneumograph
Pneumotachometer/graph
Pop-off valve
Pressure regulator
Pressure relief valve
Pulse monitor
Pulse rate meter
Rebreathing bag
Rebreathing circuit
Rees T-piece paediatric circuit
Regulator
Reservoir bag
Respirable air pump
Respirator
Respirometer
Resuscitator
Rocking apparatus
Rotameter
Ruben's valve
Salt valve
Scavenging system
Schimmelbusch mask
Semi-closed circuit
Spirometer/spirograph
Suction catheter
Suction machine
T-piece circuit
Tracheostomy tube
Ultrasonic nebulizer
Vacuum control valve
Vacuum pump
Vacuum unit
Vaporizer
Venous pressure monitor
Ventilator
Ventilator alarm
Vital signs monitor
Wall suction unit
Waters canister
Williams filter
Wright's respiration monitor/meter
Wright's respirometer

Entries relevant to audiology and speech therapy

Acoustic booth
Acoustic impedance meter/bridge
Anechoic chamber
Artificial ear
Artificial larynx
Artificial mastoid
Audiometer
Auriscope
Averager
Barany box
Bekesy audiometer
Bone conduction transducer/
  receiver
Bone vibrator
Caloric apparatus
Cochlea implant
Delayed auditory feedback
  machine
Ear mould
Edinburgh masker
Electret microphone
Electric response audiometer
Electro-aerometer
Electrocochleograph
Electroglottograph
Electrogustometer
Electronystagmograph (ENG)
Evoked response averager
Exeter lip sensor
Exeter visual speech aid
Free-field audiometer
Frenzel glasses
Glottograph
Grommet
Headphone
Hearing aid
Hearing aid test box
Inductive loop
Infrared viewer
Laryngograph
Laryngoscope
Masker
Myophone
Nasal anemometer
Nystagmograph
Octave band analyser
Optokinetic drum
Otoacoustic emission processor/

audiometer
Otoscope
Phonic ear
Phonic mirror
Pistonphone
Pure tone audiometer
Relaxometer
Screening audiometer
Siegles speculum
Sona-graph
Sound level meter
Spectrascribe
Spectrograph/spectroscope
Speech amplifier
Speech audiometer
Speech synthesizer
Speech trainer
Stimulator
Tinnitus masker
Tuning fork
Tympanometer
Voiscope
Warble-tone audiometer
Wax bath

Entries relevant to cardiology

Ambulatory ECG monitor
Arrhythmia detector
Ballistocardiograph
Cardiac angiography apparatus
Cardiac catheterization equipment
Cardiac microphone
Cardiac output computer
Cardiac pacemaker
Cardioscope
Cardiotachometer
Cardioverter
Defibrillator
Dye dilution computer
ECG monitor
Echocardiograph
Electrical impedance cardiac out-
  put computer
Electrocardiograph
Ergometric recording system
Fibre-optic recorder
Fibrillator
Fick cardiac output computer
Floating electrode

Flow-directed catheter
Heart rate meter
His bundle analyser
Impedance plethysmograph
Intra-aortic balloon
M-mode (ultrasonic) scanner
Monitored defibrillator
Oesophageal pacemaker
Pacemaker
Pacemaker analyser
Phased array (ultrasonic) scanner
Phonocardiograph
Phonocatheter
Spirometer/spirograph
Stethoscope
Stimulator
Suction electrode
Swan-Ganz catheter
Telemetry
Thermodilution cardiac output
    computer
Time-motion (TM) scanner
Treadmill
Trend recorder
Vectorcardiograph

Entries relevant to dialysis

Air embolus detector
Arteriovenous shunt
Artificial kidney
Blood leak detector
Blood level detector
Blood pump
Bubble trap
Conductivity meter
Continuous ambulatory peritoneal
    dialysis (CAPD)
De-aerator
De-ionizer
Dialysate conductivity meter
Dialysate pressure monitor
Dialysate proportionating pump
Dialyser
Dialyser washout device
Dialysis clamp
Fistula monitor
Haemodialysis machine
Haemofiltration apparatus
Haemoheater
Haemoperfusion apparatus

Heparin pump
Peristaltic pump
Peritoneal dialysis clamp
Peritoneal dialysis machine
Proportioning pump
Pump
Reverse osmosis machine
Roller pump
Single-needle device
Ultrafiltration apparatus
Ultrafiltration monitor
Water softener

Entries relevant to electronics, computers and equipment servicing

ADC/DAC interface
Antistatic chain
Antistatic floor
Antistatic rubber
Auto-transformer
Averager
Bi-stable storage cathode ray tube
    (CRT)
Cathode ray tube
Chart recorder
Computer
Constant voltage transformer
Defibrillator tester
Diathermy tester
Differential amplifier
Earth leakage circuit breaker
    (ELCB)
Earth leakage current meter/
    monitor
Earth loop tester
Electrode
Faraday cage
Flatbed recorder
FM tape recorder
Impedance bridge
Ink-jet recorder
Integrator
Isolating transformer
Leakage current monitor
Light pen
Linear variable differential transformer (LVDT)
Load cell transducer
Memory oscilloscope
Microelectrode

Modem
Neutral electrode
Oscilloscope
Patient circuit
Pattern generator
Potentiometric recorder
Storage cathode ray tube
Strain gauge transducer
Tape recorder
Thermistor
Thermocouple
Thermometer
Transducer
Transient recorder
Trend recorder
Ultraviolet recorder
Visual display unit
$X-Y$ recorder

Entries relevant to lung function testing

Absorption spectrometer
Body box
Capnometer/capnograph
Carbon dioxide analyser
Carbon monoxide analyser
Emission spectroscope
Fleisch tube
Functional residual capacity (FRC) analyser
Helium dilution (FRC) analyser
Infrared carbon dioxide analyser
Katharometer
Nitrogen analyser
Peak flowmeter
Pneumograph
Pneumotachometer/graph
Spirometer/spirograph
Transfer factor analyser
Vitalograph
Wright peak flowmeter

Entries relevant to ionizing radiation

Applicator
Ardran–Crooks cassette
Arterio-angiography apparatus
Auto-gamma counter

Beta counter
Betatron
Bucky diaphragm
Cardiac angiography apparatus
CAT scanner
Cineangiography apparatus
Cobalt-60 treatment unit
Collimator
Coolidge tube
CT scanner
Densitometer
Dose-rate meter
Dosemeter/dosimeter
EMI scanner
Emission tomography (ECAT) scanner
Film badge
Film changer
Fluoroscope
Gamma camera
Geiger–Müller tube
Grentz-ray set
Hardening filter
Image intensifier
Ionization chamber
Ionizing radiation
Isotope cow
Isotope scanner
kV_p meter
Light beam diaphragm
Linear accelerator
Liquid scintillation counter
Mammography system
Multichannel analyser
Orthovoltage X-ray set
Penetrameter
Phantom
Photomultiplier (PM) tube
Potter-bucky diaphragm
Pulse height analyser
Radiotherapy equipment
Radium needle
Radium tube
Rectilinear scanner
Scintillation camera
Scintillation counter
Sealed source
Sensitometer
Spectrograph/spectroscope
Spinning top
Step wedge

283

Superficial X-ray treatment unit
Teleisotope unit
Teletherapy apparatus
Thermoluminescent dosimetry
  apparatus
Tomographic X-ray unit
Well counter
Wisconsin test cassette
Xeroradiography apparatus
X-ray film cassette
X-ray set
X-ray therapy apparatus
X-ray tube

**Entries relevant to medical
  laboratories**

Atomic absorption spectrometer
Auto analyser
Beta counter
Blood gas analyser
Centrifuge
Centrifugal analyser
Chart recorder
Chromatograph
Colorimeter
Continuous flow analyser
Coulter counter
Cuvette
Densitometer
Discrete sample analyser
Electrophoresis apparatus
Enzyme analyser
Flame photometer
Fluorescence spectrometer
Fluorimeter (fluorometer)
Gas–liquid chromatograph (GLC)
Haematocrit centrifuge
Haemacytometer/haemocytometer
Incubator
Ion selective electrode
Liquid scintillation counter
Mass spectroscope/spectrograph
Microtome
Monochromator
Multichannel analyser
Nephelometer
Oil heating bath
Osmometer
pH meter
Photometer

Potassium ion analyser
Proportioning pump
Reaction rate analyser
Shaker
Spectrophotometer
Stat analyser
Stirrer
Turbidimeter
Water bath

Miscellaneous items

Acupuncture apparatus
Air bed
Apnoea alarm/monitor
Applanation tonometer
Arteriosonde
Autoclave
Babywarmer
Bed weighing system
Biofeedback apparatus
Bladder stimulator
Blood flow meter
Blood pressure monitor/meter
Blood velocity meter
Blood warmer
Breast pump
Carbon dioxide cystometer
Cardiff infusion system
Cardiotocograph
Cast cutter
Catheter puller
Catholysis unit
Chart recorder
Checkerboard stimulator
Chemical thermometer
Clark electrode
Cystometer
Depilator
Drop counter/ratemeter
Drop detector head
Electrical stimulator
Electroconvulsive therapy
  apparatus
Electrode
Electroencephalograph (EEG)
Electrolysis unit
Electromyograph (EMG)
Electronarcosis apparatus
Electronystagmograph (ENG)
Electro-oculograph

Electroretinograph
Electrosleep apparatus
Endoradiosonde
Epilation unit
Evoked response averager
Eye magnet
Flatbed recorder
Floating electrode
Flow-directed catheter
Foetal electrocardiograph
Foetal heart detector
Foetal monitor/recorder
Fogging machine
Force plate/platform
Formalin sterilizing unit/cabinet
Fumigation unit
Functional electrical stimulator
  (FES)
Galvanometric recorder
Ganzfeld stimulator
Gastric pump
Goniometer
Guard ring tocograph
Gustometer
Haemoheater
Haemotonometer
Heart-assist device
Heart–lung machine
Heart simulator
Heat camera
Heated gloves/socks
Heated ripple mattress
Heating bath
Hyperbaric therapy apparatus
Impedance plethysmograph
Incubator
Inductive loop
Infrared camera
Infrared lamp
Infusion controller
Infusion pump
Integrator
Intra-aortic balloon
Iontophoresis apparatus
Kymograph
Mercury manometer
Mercury plethysmograph
Microelectrode
Motorized syringe
MR scanner
Nasal anemometer

Nerve stimulator
Nuclear magnetic resonance
  (NMR) scanner
Nystagmograph
Ophthalmodynamometer
Ophthalmometer
Ophthalmoscope
Orthosis
Otoscope
Overhead baby warmer
Oximeter
Oxygen concentrator
Pasteurizer
Pattern generator
Perimeter
Peripheral nerve stimulator
Peristaltic pump
Phonophoresis apparatus
Photic stimulator
Photometer
Photoplethysmograph
Phototherapy apparatus
Piped vacuum service
Plethysmograph
Pneumograph
Polarographic cell
Polygraph
Pressure transducer
Profilometer
Prosthesis
Pulse duplicator
Pulse monitor
Pulse rate meter
Pump
Pupillometer
Puva skin treatment apparatus
Radiation thermometer
Radio pill
Retinoscope
Ripple bed/mattress
Skin resistance meter
Slit lamp
Sphygmomanometer
Sterilizer
Sterotoner
Stethoscope
Stimulator
Stomach pump
Suction catheter
Suction machine
Syringe pump

$TcpO_2$ monitor
Telemetry
Thermocouple
Thermograph
Thermometer
Tocodynamometer
Tonometer
Tourniquet
Transcutaneous electrical neural
   stimulator (TENS)
Transducer
Ultrasonic nebulizer
Urilos electronic nappy
Urinometer
Urodynamic apparatus
Uroflowmeter
Vacuum pump
Vascular dilator
Venous occlusion plethysmograph
Venous pressure monitor
Visual field analyser
Vocoder
Volumetric infusion pump
Walking platform
Water bed/mattress
Water manometer
Weighing bed

Entries relevant to physiotherapy

Actinotherapy apparatus
Acupuncture apparatus
Cryotherapy apparatus
Current bath
Diathermy equipment
Dynamometer
Electrotherapy apparatus
Faradic treatment unit
Heatlamp
Heat treatment unit
Hot pack heater
Hydrocollator pack
Hydrotherapy apparatus
Inductothermy apparatus
Infrared lamp
Interferential treatment unit
Intermittent compression
   apparatus
Kromayer lamp
Microwave diathermy apparatus
Phototherapy apparatus

Progressive treatment unit
Radiant heat lamp
Short-wave diathermy apparatus
Smart Bristow faradic coil
Stimulator
Suction therapy apparatus
Theraktin tunnel bath
Therapeutic diathermy equipment
Traction apparatus
Tunnel bath
Ultrasonic diathermy apparatus
Ultrasonic massager
Ultrasonic transducer
Ultrasonic treatment unit
Ultraviolet treatment lamp
Vibromassager
Wax bath
Whirlpool bath

Entries relevant to surgery

Active electrode
Air embolus detector
Arthroscope
Artificial artery
Artificial heart
Artificial heart valve
Bipolar coagulator
Bipolar surgical diathermy
Blood loss meter
Bone saw
Bronchoscope
Bubble oxygenator
Bubble trap
Carbon dioxide insufflation
   apparatus
Cardiopulmonary bypass apparatus
Cautery unit
Cold light source
Colonoscope
Colposcope
Cryosurgery apparatus
Culdoscope
Cystoscope
Diathermy equipment
Dispersive electrode
Electrocautery apparatus
Electromagnetic blood flowmeter
Electrosurgery unit
Endoscope
Fibre-optic light source

Flexoplate
Flexoplate monitor
Gastroscope
Goniometer
Hyfrecator
Indifferent electrode
Insufflation apparatus
Laser (surgical)
Light plethysmograph
Lithotriptor
Metal fragment detector
Nephroscope
Neutral electrode
Oscillating saw
Oxygenator
Panendoscope
Perometer
Plasma scalpel
Proctoscope
Prosthesis
Roller pump
Sigmoidoscope
Suction catheter
Surgical diathermy machine
Urethroscope
Xenograft

**Entries relevant to medical
ultrasound**

A-scanner
AIUM test object
Arteriosonde
B-scanner
Bi-stable storage cathode ray tube
  (CRT)
C-scanner (ultrasonic)
Calipers (ultrasonic)
Calorimeter
Compound (ultrasonic) scanner
Doppler blood flow/velocity meter
Doppler foetal heart detector/
  monitor
Doppler (ultrasonic) blood
  pressure monitor
Doppler ultrasonic scanner

Echocardiograph
Echoencephalograph
Fibre-optic recorder
Foetal heart detector
Frame-freeze module
Grey scale display unit
Light pen
Linear array (ultrasound) scanner
M-mode (ultrasonic) scanner
Mavis (Movable Arterial and
  Venous Imaging System)
Midliner
Multiformat camera
Octoson
Phantom
Phased array (ultrasonic) scanner
Plan position indicator (ultrasonic)
  scanner
Pulsed wave doppler ultrasonic
  flowmeter
Radiation pressure (force) balance
Range-gated doppler ultrasonic
  flowmeter
Real-time ultrasonic scanner
Scan converter
Section (ultrasound) scanner
Spectrograph/spectroscope
Step wedge
Stop-action (ultrasonic) scanner
Time compression analyser
Time–motion (TM) scanner
Transcutaneous aortic velograph
  (TAV)
Transmission-mode (ultrasonic)
  scanner
Ultrasonic blood flow rate meter
Ultrasonic blood pressure monitor
Ultrasonic cleaning bath
Ultrasonic diathermy apparatus
Ultrasonic massager
Ultrasonic nebulizer
Ultrasonic scanner
Ultrasonic stethoscope
Ultrasonic transducer
Ultrasonic treatment unit
Zero-crossing ratemeter

Appendix 3

Reference literature (as code (r) with each item)

1. McDicken, W.N.(1981) *Diagnostic Ultrasonics:Principles and Use of Instruments,* 2nd edn, John Wiley and Sons, New York.

2. Ward, C.S.(1975) *Anaesthetic Equipment: Physical Principles and Maintenance,* Bailliere Tyndall, 7 and 8 Henrietta Street, London WC2E 8QE.

3. Brown, B.H. and Smallwood, R.H.(1981) *Medical Physics and Physiological Measurement,* Blackwell Scientific Publications, Osney Mead, Oxford OX2 0EL, UK.

4. Cook, A.M. and Webster, J.G. (1982) *Therapeutic Medical Devices: Application and Design,* Prentice-Hall Inc., Englewood Cliffs, NJ 07632, USA.

5. Ackerman, P.G. (1972) *Electronic Instrumentation in the Clinical Laboratory,* Little, Brown and Co., Boston, Mass., USA.

6. Hill, D.W. and Dolan, A.M. (1982) *Intensive Care Instrumentation,* 2nd edn, Academic Press Inc.(London) Ltd., 24/28 Oval Road, London NW1, UK, and Grune and Stratten Inc., 111 Fifth Avenue, New York, NY, 10003.

7. Van der Plaats, G.J. (1980) *Medical and X-ray Techniques in Diagnostic Radiology,* 4th edn, The Macmillan Press Ltd., London.

8. Burns, W. (1973) *Noise and Man,* 2nd edn, John Murray, 50 Albemarle Street, London.

9. Webster, John G.(Ed.) (1978) *Medical Instrumentation: Application and Design,* Houghton Mifflin Company, Boston, Dallas, Geneva, Illinois, Hopewell, New Jersey, Palo Alto, London.

10. Forster, Angela and Palastanga, Nigel, (1981) *Clayton's Electrotherapy,* 8th edn, Bailliere Tindall, 7 and 8 Henrietta Street, London WC2E 8QE.